The Patient Advoc

300 Questions And Answers
To Help You Care For Your Loved One

At the Hospital And At Home

This handbook discusses common situations created by illness and recovery to offer you relevant and practical information ahead of time, so your increased familiarity with healthcare issues will lead to better results for your loved one. Keep this handbook with you to optimize the hospital stay and have a more effective and less stressful experience with your loved one's home care.

~~~~~~

"I am confident that this book will be an invaluable reference and resource for families and caregivers. Perhaps more importantly, I know it will provide a measure of reassurance to those facing seemingly insurmountable health challenges that they are not powerless – and they certainly are not alone."

Jon Kobashigawa MD

Clinical Professor of Medicine
The David Geffen School of Medicine
University of California at Los Angeles

Director, Center for Advanced Heart Disease
Director, Heart Transplant Program
Cedars-Sinai Heart Institute

"Kudos for an outstanding book to inform patient advocates confronted with a dizzying and perplexing array of issues within our current health system. It is a very good idea and much needed."

Elias Zerhouni MD
Former Director, National Institutes of Health
Bethesda, Maryland

~~~~~~

"Outstanding! I found the information to be very credible, easy to read and very informative. It will help countless families as they care for their loved ones."

David T. Feinberg MD MBA
CEO UCLA Hospital System
Associate Vice Chancellor

~~~~~~

"A rare compendium crafted with care and compassion. An essential guide to navigating the complexities of home care."

Peter C. Whybrow MD
Director, Semel Institute for Neuroscience
and Human Behavior
Judson Braun Distinguished Professor and Executive Chair
Department of Psychiatry and Biobehavioral Sciences
at the David Geffen School of Medicine at UCLA
Physician-In-Chief, Resnick Neuropsychiatric Hospital

"The suggestions on working with hospital inpatient staff, coordinating homecare and understanding the complexities of Medicare and private insurance make for excellent content. The short question and succinct declarative answer format makes it easy for someone to scan the book for a topic of interest."

Thomas Strouse MD
Medical Director
Stewart and Lynda Resnick Neuropsychiatric Hospital
at UCLA
Professor of Clinical Psychiatry
David Geffen-UCLA School of Medicine

~~~~~~

"This is a very valuable resource for patients' families that will bring practical guidance and peace of mind to them."

Laurence Marton MD
Former Dean, University of Wisconsin School of Medicine

~~~~~~

"I like the question/answer format. It's very accessible and easy to follow and is a breakthrough in a "user's guide" in the medical area."

Mary Woolley PhD
President, Research!America
Alexandria, VA

Foreword

In my twenty-three years as a cardiologist, I have worked with countless families striving to navigate the complex challenges of caring for a critically ill loved one. In that time, I have met few more dedicated and caring than Jim Williams and his family.

I first met Jim in April of 2004 when his mother, Jane, suffered a devastating stroke. Jim and his father devoted their lives to Jane's care for the next 3 ½ years, learning to manage every aspect of her medical treatment during subsequent hospital stays and home recovery. Her quality of life during this difficult time was in large part due to their constant diligence and intensity of focus.

As with many families in similar situations, the Williams family found themselves in unfamiliar territory, making decisions under tremendous pressure, often with limited information. Jim and his family did their utmost to learn from and cooperate with doctors and nurses, proactively finding creative ways to help Jane cope and improve – a true testament to their commitment and resolve.

The lessons they learned as Jane's condition took its course were hard earned. These serve as the foundation of this remarkable book, unique in its wealth of practical solutions for many of the most common situations and decisions facing advocates of loved ones in need of ongoing medical care at the hospital and assistance at home.

It contains useful tips and advice relating to stroke and rehabilitation, but most of the issues addressed are not necessarily disease, affliction or even age-specific. They can be applied to a wide range of conditions requiring acute care, including elective surgery, "elderly diseases" like stroke, cancer and Alzheimer's and those faced mostly by younger patients from trauma due to auto and motorcycle accidents as well as athletic injuries.

After 3 ½ years of actively participating in his mother's care, Jim spent another 2 years writing and polishing this book into its present form: a user friendly, practical handbook for advocates. It is indeed well named.

I am confident that this book will be an invaluable reference and resource for families and caregivers. Perhaps more importantly, I know it will provide a measure of reassurance to those facing seemingly insurmountable health challenges that they are not powerless – and they certainly are not alone.

Jon Kobashigawa MD

Clinical Professor of Medicine
The David Geffen School of Medicine
University of California at Los Angeles

Director, Center for Advanced Heart Disease
Director, Heart Transplant Program
Cedars-Sinai Heart Institute

Preface

I wrote The Patient Advocate's Handbook to help you care for your loved one by organizing what I learned as an advocate into a handy reference, so you can quickly deal with common healthcare issues.

I wish I had this handbook during the 3 ½ years I assisted my father in the care of my mother. With each new issue, we struggled to find solutions and hoped we had made the right decisions. This book pre-packages much of the basic, but overwhelming details commonly faced by advocates to provide you with concise explanations, options and suggestions.

This book is not a "disease book"; it is an advocacy book. A disease book examines the disease itself; it's causes, progression, treatments and potential complications. It is not an examination of emotional/psychological caregiving issues and is not an encyclopedia of bedside care. This book will help you be a better advocate sooner in the process by describing common situations and giving you practical options no matter the cause of the medical condition.

I would also like to mention that I am not a medical professional and I have no interest, financial ownership or agreement with any healthcare entity. My motivation is to give you the benefit of my experience to help you become the best advocate you can be.

James Thomas Williams

The
Patient Advocate's
Handbook

300 Questions And Answers
To Help You Care For Your Loved One

At The Hospital And At Home

James Thomas Williams

Panglossian Press
Los Angeles, California

The Patient Advocate's Handbook
300 Questions And Answers
To Help You Care For Your Loved One
At The Hospital And At Home

ISBN: 978-0-9842825-0-0

LCCN: 2009943230

Panglossian Press
14006 Palawan Way, suite 315
Los Angeles, California 90292

www.thepatientadvocateshandbook.com

Internet addresses cited in the book and its appendices
were verified as of December, 2009.

Contents

This Book Is Organized To Save Time

As an advocate, you are feeling stressed, overtired, rushed and overwhelmed. This handbook is designed with the following features for quick reference:

Question/answer format
The book is organized in a concise question/answer format, so you can easily see questions posed, suggestions offered and find closely related questions and suggestions.

Detailed Table of Contents
Chapters and their subheadings organize the Table of Contents. Scan for topics described by the subheadings and go to a topic page for relevant questions and suggestions.

Chapter introductions
Each chapter starts with a single page summary. Read all of them at the outset to become familiar with the purpose of each chapter. This will help you think ahead and plan effectively as your loved one moves from hospital to home.

Internal page references
Many topics have references to other pages where a term is discussed in relation to another topic for definition or elaboration.

Questions are listed for browsing
Appendix 11 lists over 300 questions sorted by chapter, subheading and page number for browsing and lookup.

Indexed keywords
Use the Index to look up topics and suggestions by indexed keyword.

To my Mother and Father

Chapter 1

At The Hospital

Mom was sitting in a wheelchair and needed to be transferred back to bed for a nap. Because she could not get up on her own, the hospital "lift team" was called to the room to move her. The guy who showed up was built like an Olympic weightlifter, a mini-Arnold Schwarzenegger. He leaned over Mom, who was 5'-7" and about 125 pounds and started to lift her up. After much straining, he wheezed, "She is really heavy. I'm not sure if I can do this." I noticed the wheelchair wheels were a few inches off the floor, so I suggested he put her down and try again after releasing the wheelchair seat belt. We all had a good laugh.

If you are caring for a loved one who is ill, you will have many new experiences as a patient advocate. At first, you may know little about how the medical system works and what you can do to help care for your loved one, but by observing and learning, trusting your instincts, applying common sense and speaking up, you will make helpful contributions to your loved one's care. As you navigate the medical journey with your loved one through the hospital and later at home, you will naturally develop knowledge and skills to become a more effective advocate.

This handbook accelerates your healthcare orientation by examining common situations, so you can be prepared sooner to participate more effectively as an advocate at the hospital and at home.

This chapter covers the hospital stay. Chapters 2, 3 and 4 bring up home healthcare issues you should consider and address before leaving the hospital.

What Is An Advocate?

I don't know what an advocate does at the hospital.

As an advocate, you will be watching over your loved one to optimize care and minimize mistakes. You'll be meeting with attending doctors and nurses to understand medical treatment recommendations and participate in medical decisions. You'll also learn from medical professionals how to observe your loved one, so you can make a more effective contribution to your loved one's care at the hospital and later at home.

What does it mean to "optimize care"?

To optimize means to make something the best it can be. You can help by speaking with health professionals to learn about available treatment alternatives and help your loved one communicate, understand and cope with an often confusing and fearful process. You can help maximize the care your loved one receives by preventing medical mistakes or neglect. You can even look into the state of research for your loved one's illness (Appendices 8 and 9).

I'm not a medical professional and I have never done this before, so I am feeling alone and helpless.

Everyone who becomes an advocate feels this way, but by taking on this responsibility, you are being of great help to your loved one. Remember, the outcome is beyond your control. Do your best and accept that there is much in the universe beyond your power and that of medical science.

At the hospital, I have moments when I get anxious and upset.

This is a normal and sometimes frequent reaction to a loved one's hospitalization. When possible, ask a friend or relative who is visiting to fill in, so you can leave to get some quiet time. Find a quiet area and listen to soothing music with a pair of earphones to keep out interfering sounds. Put your cell phone on vibrate mode and hold it on your hand, so you won't miss a call from a doctor or the person relieving you. Don't use meal times in the cafeteria or sitting in the waiting room as your only time away from your loved one's room.

I feel guilty because I can't be there 24 hours a day.

No one can, so don't make the common mistake of staying at the hospital until you're physically and mentally exhausted. Once the initial period of admission, diagnosis and treatment decision is past, ask a family member or friend to fill in, so you can get some rest. They will call if they need you.

I am frustrated and afraid.

You may feel like you are being manipulated by the "system" and become angry, frustrated and afraid, but don't let it get the better of you. Never lose your temper and act out your negative feelings. Never threaten to sue. Those who witness your hostility will no longer want to deal with you. While you may feel better after your outburst, those on the receiving end might tell others about the incident, causing them to shun you as well.

Going To The Hospital

What if I need to transport my loved one to a hospital?

Non-emergencies
If the trip to the hospital is not an emergency, but is medically necessary and your loved one is considered "homebound" (page 57) by Medicare (leaving the home requires considerable and taxing effort), Medicare and insurance may cover most of the cost for private ambulance transport to the hospital and for the return trip home. This must be pre-arranged with a prescription from the doctor to a private ambulance company, not by calling 911.

Emergencies
If the trip to the hospital is an emergency, call 911 and they (usually Fire Department paramedics) will take your loved one to the closest emergency room (ER). If they are going with "lights and siren", getting your loved one to the closest ER is a top priority. Don't ask to go to a more distant hospital ER.

Ask the paramedics where they plan to take your loved one. If your loved one seems stable and alert to the paramedics, it is possible the paramedics will consider taking your loved one to an ER you prefer (for example, at your loved one's hospital) if it is no more than a couple of miles or a few additional minutes further away than the closest ER. Ask them if your loved one's condition and their caseload will allow them to travel a few extra minutes. If you don't bring it up, you'll never know. They don't have to do favors, so if they don't think your request is the best way, accept their answer without question.

Transport between hospitals
After your loved one has been stabilized at the closest ER, critical care ambulance transport to the another hospital may be necessary for further treatment. The transport is arranged by the sending and receiving hospitals and must be medically

necessary for Medicare and insurance to consider covering it.

<u>Information To Have Ready</u>

What information should I keep available to offer to healthcare professionals?

For ambulance transport (emergency, non-emergency and critical care), the emergency room (ER), hospital admissions and doctors and nurses, keep handy copies of your loved one's:

Medicare card
Supplemental (Medi-Gap) card
Private insurance card

Medical History	(below)
Medicines List	(page 6)
Medicine Chart	(page 6)
Side Effects/Allergies List	(page 6)
Advance Directives	(page 7)
Doctor Information List	(page 8)

What is a Medical History?

This is a historical recitation of medical events leading up to the current condition. Include doctor names and specialties, medical conditions and diseases. While it may not be the direct cause of the current hospital visit, a medical condition or disease could have a bearing on the treatment or the ability of your loved one to cope and recover. Include "assisting" devices like a pacemaker (a medical device using electrical impulses, delivered by electrodes contacting the heart muscles, to regulate the beating of the heart).

What is a Medicines List?

It's a list of medicines ordered, the ordering doctors, specified dosages and the number of times to be given per day. It also lists over the counter (OTC) medicines and supplements. It includes medicines given in the past, which were discontinued by order of the doctor or ended like a temporary course (prescribed duration) of an antibiotic.

What is a Medicine Chart?

This record of prescribed medicines is updated with each dose given and each dose held (not given per doctor's order or nurse discretion). It also notes discontinued medicines. At the hospital, doctors and nurses can review your entries in your loved one's home Medicine Chart (Appendix 3) to see what was given at home.

What is a Side Effects/Allergies List?

This should be at the top of the Medicines List. It includes anything that produced a side effect or an allergic reaction, the effect or reaction and what was done about it. Was a substance discontinued and if so, what was used instead?

My loved one has an allergy to a medicine. How can I be sure this medicine will not be given?

At arrival, you'll fill out standard patient information forms. Either the hospital has a record of your loved one from a previous stay and will need to update their records or they will create a new record on the first visit. The hospital will print out the updated record for you to examine and sign. Be sure it specifically lists all allergies and there are no inaccurate inclusions. (In our case, Mom was not diabetic,

but the updated form printout said, "Patient is diabetic".)
Be sure information from past visits is still included in the
updated record and none has been mistakenly deleted. (Mom
had a pacemaker and the updated printout had no mention
of it.)

Write inaccuracies on the updated record and ask the
admissions person to correct them and then carefully RE-
EXAMINE the revised printout! Once you are satisfied the
information is accurate and up to date, it will be used to
generate accurate hospital records, charts, labels and patient
wristbands.

**Is there anything in addition I can do to minimize
medicinal allergy mistakes?**

Ask a nurse to show you the allergy entry is also included in
the bedside chart. In addition, mention the allergy to nurses
who are seeing your loved one for the first time. Also, post a
large notice in the hospital room where everyone will see it,
such as "Allergic to ..."

What are Advance Directives?

Advance Directives are written instructions regarding your
loved one's medical care preferences, including a Living Will,
a Medical Power of Attorney and a Do Not Resuscitate Order
(DNS). The family and medical professionals will consult
these instructions if a loved one is unable to make health
care decisions.

For in-depth explanations of advance directives:

http://www.mayoclinic.com/health/living-wills/HA00014

What information should I be gathering to refer to in the future?

While at the hospital and later at home, start building and continue to add to these lists (keep them readily available):

Hospital Information List
This list (Appendix 1) makes it easier to find and remember hospital locations and tell visitors how to find your loved one. It includes directions to the ER, parking structure, hospital admissions office and your loved one's unit or room.

Doctor Information List
This list (Appendix 1) is a sub-section of the Hospital Information List and includes the names and contact information of doctors and nurses who have been and are involved with your loved one's case. The information is useful to health care professionals, for example ER doctors, who may want to consult with other doctors to gain a more complete understanding of your loved one's medical condition. You may not be able to recall this information while under stress, so keep this updated list with you.

Home Healthcare Contact Information List
This list (Appendix 2) includes phone numbers and Internet addresses of home healthcare supply companies, Internet vendors, mobile X-ray companies and visiting nurses. Include the private insurance customer service manager's and group administrator's names and phone numbers.

Why should I also keep the insurance customer service and group administrator information with me?

If there is a question about coverage, you may need to call

customer service to get clarification or correct a mistake. If your loved one has been accidentally "termed out" (cancelled by mistake) of insurance coverage, you'll need to call an administrator to be "re-instated" (resume coverage).

Gathering And Sharing Information

What is the "Chimney Effect" and what can I do about it?

This expression refers to the flow of information. You can count on information (smoke) to travel naturally up a medical specialty hierarchy (chimney), but not to be shared as quickly or reliably across disciplines (separate chimneys). Because medical conditions change, you should assist as much as you can, so the latest information is fully shared as quickly as possible.

How can I help move information along?

Information must be accurate, complete and quickly shared to be meaningful. Make notes about discussions and include doctor names as well as times and dates. Ask the doctor which other doctors are involved and list the questions to ask them. Double-check later with the primary doctor to close the loop regarding information relayed to you, decisions made and any changed or new orders.

What about technology and the computerization of medical records?

Computerized records are created for easy reference, but the original information must be valid and then the person must input it into the database without errors or omissions. No technology can replace you and your dedication to the timeliness of accurate information. Anytime you see a computer record of your loved one, examine it with a critical eye. This includes hospital information records and charts, both printed and on-screen, as well as medical insurance statements.

Information Privacy

Could privacy issues get in the way?

The Health Insurance Portability and Accountability Act (HIPAA) governs patient privacy and limits disclosure of "Individually Identifiable Health Information" to certain individuals, including one's family and friends, regardless of one's state of health. If you are not authorized under HIPAA to discuss a patient's private matters with doctors and nurses and view charts and records, ask the hospital about release forms. For example, a HIPPA Privacy Release is required to be signed by the patient or by a legally designated person authorized to sign legal documents on behalf of the patient.

What about HIPAA and emergencies?

HIPAA does not prevent a health professional from discussing care if it's in the best interest of the patient, for example to help a doctor in an emergency situation.

The Effective Advocate

Everyone says advocates are needed, but do doctors and nurses really want advocates?

Doctors and nurses need effective advocates whose relevant input is helpful in the delivery of effective care. Nurses are trained to be patient advocates and you can expect them to welcome an advocacy relationship with you, so don't be shy about speaking up. Share your concerns and suggestions and ask their opinions. If you provide information about the medical condition of your loved one or prevent or discover a mistake, you will help the situation. But, if you panic, express anger and frustration or are indiscrete or impolite, you can diminish the care of your loved one by obstructing, distracting or alienating the medical team.

What best describes an "effective" advocate?

An effective advocate asks questions, learns how to observe and understands the importance remaining emotionally steady and polite when faced with uncertainty and stress.

Because I am not a medical professional and I am emotionally involved, won't I be forgiven for under or over reacting to a given situation?

If you under reacted, forgiveness has to come from within. You didn't speak up or push your concerns enough at the time and now, that time is past. You can't spend your energy regretting what you should have done.

If you over reacted, admit it. But, if you also lost your cool, panicked and were abusive or arrogant, those on the receiving end of your tirade will no longer want you as part of the process. Make a sincere apology, but until things cool off, another person should speak to the medical team on your behalf.

I don't know what you mean by "under reacting".

Here are three common ways people under react to their loved one's needs and how you can prevent it:

You don't realize something is wrong, because you don't know what to watch for.
Learn from health professionals how to observe your loved one and ask them what to watch for. Learning about your loved one's condition and care involves asking many questions. As an advocate, you have a right to learn how you can be helpful in watching over and caring for your loved one.

You sense there is a problem, but you don't want to be pushy, so you don't speak up.
If you have a specific concern, speak with a nurse or doctor right away! Also, don't wait for problems to arise to ask general questions to help you learn about your loved one's medical condition and treatment.

You sense there is a problem and speak up, but no one double-checks thoroughly and you don't pursue it further, because you don't know who to approach and specifically what to ask for.
Start with the attending nurse and move up the chain of command until you feel informed and reassured. If you are not satisfied your concern has been addressed, speak with the doctor.

The following topics will help you become better at observing your loved one at the hospital and asking relevant questions of health professionals. Also explained are diplomatic ways to mention your concerns as well as what you can do to follow up.

<u>Learning To Observe</u>

I'm in intensive care with my loved one, but I don't know what is important to observe and pay attention to.

In an intensive care unit, there is a critical care nurse near the bed, so your value as an advocate is mainly to discuss treatment. You have an opportunity in this very supportive setting to ask about what to observe.

How will I know what to observe?

Ask about the purpose of medical equipment connected to your loved one. Medical equipment has warning messages and alarms, so ask what they mean. Some are set to a high sensitivity to indicate even a mild abnormality, like an irregular heartbeat, which may be normal for your loved one. Once you understand which are routine alarms and messages (occurring the most often), you can be alert for more serious ones (occurring less often). When you ask questions to become familiar with the hospital environment, always try to use a calm tone of voice or the nurse might mistakenly believe there is a serious problem.

In intensive care, nurses and doctors are always near my loved one's bed, so why should I care about what to observe?

Each day in the hospital with your loved one can make you a more effective advocate. Stay alert and use the supportive setting of an Intensive Care Unit (ICU) to learn. After your loved one is moved from the ICU to a standard hospital room where a nurse is not always near the bed, your improved ability to observe will make you a better bedside advocate.

My loved one wasn't in intensive care before being in a hospital room, so how can I learn what to observe?

This is a less supportive setting, but you are usually watching over a much less serious situation. So relax a bit, but still ask the nurses about the equipment, connections, messages and alarms.

What is the difference with my role as an observer after my loved one moves from intensive care to a standard hospital room?

An intensive care unit has patients in critical condition in need of bedside patient monitoring to provide an instant response, whereas a hospital floor has medically stable patients in a more reactive setting where the nurse response isn't always as fast. With an increased danger from delay, mistake or neglect, a hospital room can be a hazardous place for your loved one, so it is an important time to stay by the bed, especially at night.

What kinds of patients are most in need of an advocate in a hospital room?

An elderly or fragile patient can become unstable. Some patients are unable to walk, speak or find and use the nurse call button. Many are still dependent on supplemental oxygen or have intravenous (IV) lines. Oxygen hoses can become loose or disconnected. A patient can grab an IV line and pull it out.

An alarm is repeating even though I understand from the doctor there is nothing wrong.

If a periodic sound or message indicates something considered normal, ask the doctor if the volume can be lowered so you can still easily hear it, but it is not as annoying or so disruptive to your loved one's sleep.

What would require a nurse response, without being an emergency?

If the machine message or alarm indicates a clogged or kinked tube feeding or intravenous (IV) line, summon a nurse, but don't get stressed out. If a few minutes go by, drop by the nurses' station and mention it. Other non-emergency alerts occur if the tube feeding or IV pump is beeping and flashing when a tube feeding formula bag or an IV infusion bag is depleted. The nurse might need to refill the feeding bag or set up another scheduled IV medicine, so it needs to be attended to, but it is not necessarily an emergency.

What about bloodstream connections, like intravenous (IV) lines? What do I need to observe and when do I alert a nurse?

An IV line connects to the bloodstream and has a limited useful life before it must be removed and replaced at another location or by another method. Other types of "invasive" lines, such as Peripherally Inserted Central Catheter (PICC) and Hickman lines are used for longer placement periods, but the typical IV line is used most often and has the shortest life.

Ask a nurse what to observe in assessing the line and its insertion point, which may include signs of infection: redness, warmness, discoloration, swelling, pain, extra sensitivity and fever. Ask about mechanical problems, such as a kinked, clogged, loose, leaking or disconnected line.

Changing a standard IV line is done every two or three days, but your loved one may exhibit a medical need to replace it sooner. If your loved one's blood vessels are difficult to find and there is no apparent medical indication to change the line on the third day, ask the attending nurse or doctor if the line will be left in place longer. If the nurse mentions a line (or wound dressing) needs replacing, ask when it will be done and make a note of it.

I want to be observant, but I don't want to give the impression I'm looking for problems.

Once you have asked questions and made some notes about the machines, their purposes and characteristics, practice your observations when the nurse has left the room. Don't hover near her unless you have questions at the time. During the day and when you first enter and before you leave the room, glance at each hose, tube and line, but don't be obvious about looking for things amiss.

I perceive a change in the appearance of my loved one, but everything else seems normal. Who should I ask and what should be verified?

Express your concerns to your nurse and try to be specific about the changes you are noticing. Changes can include skin color turning from normal to gray or from normal to flushed, increased facial grimacing, becoming non-responsive and changes in the breathing rate and pattern. You can ask your nurse to review medical chart entries, including:

Medicines	(being given and discontinued)
When given	(dosage times each day)
How given	(oral, injection, intravenous)
Duration of the order	(once, days, weeks, indefinite)

Nurse's notes   (daily observations)
Supplemental oxygen   (liters per minute)
Recorded vital signs   (heart rate, etc...)

Vital signs monitor
Ask the nurse to explain the readings on the vital signs
monitor, if a monitor is present. A critical care nurse told me
they are taught to "treat the patient, not the monitor", which
means they pay attention to the monitor, but use experience
and judgment to evaluate the monitor information as part
of assessment and treatment. The monitor may seem to
indicate a problem, but its information is only a part of what
the medical team will consider to decide if your loved one
needs a modification of treatment.

**If the nurse has double-checked everything, but I am
still not reassured, what can I do?**

Let your doctor know your concerns and why you want her
to get involved. The medical team might discover an error,
drug interaction or an additional medical problem. They may
decide to change some aspect of the treatment. Of course,
you hope they find nothing wrong.

Handling Yourself With Doctors And Nurses

Is there a way to stay "ahead of the curve"?

When you and your loved one arrive at a critical care unit or
a hospital floor, introduce yourself to those in charge, so later
there will be some familiarity. Don't forget substitute and
night shift charge nurses.

**My concern is a minor one, so I don't want to make
waves.**

Look to natural leaders working the unit or floor. They may not be officially in charge, but you'll recognize and feel comfortable with them because they are experienced, patient and confident. As long as you don't put them in a difficult position with their supervisors or coworkers, they will share their opinions and do what they can to help.

What can I do if I want a different nurse?

Move up the chain of command and speak with the charge nurse, then the nurse supervisor, if necessary. Always speak in the privacy of an office and politely make your case. The doctor has no official scheduling authority to make nurse assignments, but he does have influence if he needs to step in. Always keep the doctor "in the loop".

What if a nurse makes a decision to change the treatment, but doesn't consult with or inform others before or after the change was made?

This is extremely rare, but I can give an example to show how we handled it. It happened in the hospital.

A nurse practitioner (NP) is a registered nurse (RN) who may also function as a primary direct provider of health care and prescribe medications. An NP caring for Mom discontinued a prescribed antibiotic several days before it was finished without notifying the prescribing doctor, his colleagues or the family. The antibiotic had worked well before, so we wondered why she improved as usual after the antibiotic started, but began to look worse before the antibiotic finished.

I mentioned my concerns to the NP and she said she ended the antibiotic early. I asked her why she did so and why she didn't tell anyone, but she wouldn't give me a reason. I was curious if she had thought the antibiotic was ineffective, so I asked her what she planned to substitute in its place, but she had not recommended anything. She was not informative or constructive and I considered the situation serious and urgent, so I bypassed the nursing chain of command and went to our primary care doctor about it. The doctor discussed it with the nurse and ordered a full course (prescribed duration) of the same antibiotic. Mom improved as expected.

Doctor Communication Issues

A doctor I want to speak with visits mostly late at night after I leave or early in the morning before I arrive.

When you arrive, request a review of the bedside chart entries to understand the most recent data, observations and decisions of the doctors and nurses who saw your loved one while you were away. To be properly updated, ask a nurse to explain the entries to you. If a family member spent the night or you hired a night shift caregiver, debrief her in the morning.

A doctor who visits during the night is harder to reach during the day.

Write down questions, so you can recall them when you have the doctor's attention. Doctors or their colleagues will visit during the day, so be available when they are most likely to appear. Find out when the daily rounds (bedside visits) take place. It might be early mornings or late evenings. A colleague of the doctor can answer your questions or can forward your questions to the doctor.

I can't find my doctor and need to speak with her.

If you need to speak with a doctor on short notice, you can have her paged. Depending on the doctor's caseload and if she is on duty, you may be able to have a conversation by phone or in person before you leave the hospital. Don't page a doctor if it can wait. Over paging is abusive, so exercise the privilege only when absolutely necessary.

I have to leave and a discussion with the doctor can't wait. I've paged without a response so far.

Ask the charge nurse to call you when the doctor appears on rounds. You can also leave a large note taped to the door of the room, so the doctor will see it when he enters. Keep in mind everyone can see the note, so limit the content to a discussion request. Tape a copy of the note on the chart as well. Murphy's Law being what it is, the doctor will probably call you as soon as you reach the parking structure. If he is expected after hours, ask the charge nurse to pass a request to the evening charge nurse to call you at home when the doctor appears. It might be 3 A.M., so keep the phone and your notes by your bed.

I don't know when the doctor is on duty.

Ask the doctor about his usual working hours and when he fills in. You can call the doctor's office and ask when the doctor is expected to be away on vacation and who fills in. The hospital unit or floor charge nurse should be able to tell you if a doctor is on duty during the day, evening or the next morning.

I keep missing the doctor.

Speak with one of her associates. In most cases, this will provide communication either through the associate or the doctor will respond in person or by phone. Be sure to ask the associate when the doctor is most likely to be available. If you have to leave the hospital before you get a chance to speak with the doctor, give a copy of your questions to the person relieving you.

I am dissatisfied with the frequency or extent of communication.

Speak with a hospital social worker or hospital patient representative. This person may make suggestions to help you improve the communication or might make a request on your behalf for another doctor to handle your loved one's case.

Hospital Dos And Don'ts

Remember to take care of yourself.

The stress of worrying about another can run down your immune system and cause you to neglect your own health needs. Getting enough sleep is important to staying well. Keep a box of disposable surgical masks (page 42) nearby in case you feel a bit under the weather. Every year, get a flu shot.

Enforce cleanliness and keep germs from spreading.

Ask the doctor about keeping kids under 12 out of the hospital room.

Make all visitors wash their hands or use a hand sanitizer gel when entering the room.

Ask visitors if they are healthy before they enter the room.

Don't leave personal belongings in the room.

You already know about wallets, jewelry and documents, which could be lost or stolen. I am referring to other items, like cosmetics and shoes. They may not be lost or stolen. They can be accidentally thrown out, especially if you keep them in the room in a plain plastic bag. You also need to keep track of essentials like eyeglasses, hearing aids and dentures. If your loved one has to change rooms, don't forget them.

Become familiar with the state of research for your loved one's condition.

To learn more about the state of professional and researcher knowledge, consult reputable high quality websites. For example, go to National Institutes of Health (NIH), Research!America, Mayo Clinic and WebMD (Appendices 8 and 9). If you want to tell the doctor about anything you found on the Internet, mention where you got your information and print the web pages.

Don't get sick in August.

August is the peak vacation time when many senior healthcare professionals are away. Those remaining must do double duty, taking care of their normal caseload and covering for their colleagues, so in August it is harder to maintain the same level of care. July is also a tough month, especially in academic hospitals when house staff rotates and new interns and residents show up. If an elective hospital visit can wait until September, do so to better ensure all your loved one's doctors are back from their vacations.

Don't get sick on a weekend.

"Don't get sick in August, especially on a weekend" is a good adaptation. August is the toughest month and August weekends are toughest, but no matter the month, hospitals staff down on weekends. The patients aren't healthier or fewer, but the staff level is reduced anyway. Even X-rays could be harder to get on weekends, because there might be only one radiologist (a physician who specializes in diagnosing disease by obtaining and interpreting medical images) on duty. This doesn't necessarily mean you should take your loved one home on a Friday to avoid staying over the weekend, but you should expect delays, remain patient and maintain vigilance during this time.

If it's Friday, consider staying in the hospital until Monday.

If your loved one has a problem during the first weekend home, your doctor could be hard to reach. You want to avoid returning to the ER on Saturday, because it typically starts filling up by Saturday afternoon and if readmission to the hospital is necessary, it could be difficult to find an available bed. On the other hand, if your loved one is doing well at the end of the week and the doctor approves a discharge, go home before the weekend. Hospitals are places where mistakes and super bugs (antibiotic resistant infections) can harm your loved one, so leave as soon as your loved one is stable.

Stay on top of scheduled procedures.

Get procedures scheduled early in the week, because "Wednesday is the new Friday". If you are told on Monday it will be done by Wednesday, ask Tuesday morning if it is still set for the next day. If it doesn't happen on schedule, then by Wednesday afternoon you need to speak with the primary care physician, because it could slide to the following Monday.

Be wary of possible patient mix-ups.

Make sure healthcare professionals check your loved one's wristband to be sure they have the right patient. This is important for blood draws, tests, X-rays and giving medicines, especially if your loved one is sharing a room.

Ask the transport team why and where they are taking your loved one.

If your loved one is being moved from the room, ask why. If your loved one has an implanted device, is the procedure a CAT scan or an MRI? Make sure they check the wristband, so they have the right patient.

Ask about the suitability of MRI and CAT scans.

Magnetic Resonance Imaging (MRI), which uses a powerful magnetic field for medical imaging, may affect or even stop an implanted device such as a pacemaker or defibrillator, so the doctor will decide if circumstances allow an MRI. An alternative imaging technique called Computed Axial Tomography (CAT or CT scan), does not affect a pacemaker, because it uses X-rays instead of magnets. The presence of a pacemaker or any implanted device should be stated in the hospital chart along with allergies.

Ask unfamiliar persons entering the room their names, professions, who they want to see and what they want.

Health professionals and everyone else entering a hospital room are supposed to introduce themselves. If someone doesn't, ask who the individual is and what he is doing there. You gave a right to know. Write down each new name and what they tell you, so you can recall who's who. Remember, even when a familiar person enters, you have a right to ask why he is there.

Don't let anyone into the room who does not tell you everything you want to know.

She was standing just outside the hospital room door in a white laboratory coat holding a clipboard. I asked her who she was and she gave me a first name only. I asked where she was from and she answered, "Home care". The hospital has a home healthcare department to dispatch visiting nurses to homes. It took three or four more pointed questions to learn she was a commission salesperson from a home healthcare company and was there to arrange the training and rental of a home ventilator. The hospital called her company, because we used them for home oxygen equipment and supplies, but I didn't know who she was and could tell by her attitude she didn't think it mattered. I told her we would get someone else.

You have enough on your mind watching over your loved one, so don't tolerate intrusive medical device salespeople or other unauthorized visitors who want to inject themselves into your loved one's care.

Pay attention to the Foley urethral catheter and request it be removed as soon as the doctor will allow.

It's an infection threat
A Foley urethral (urine duct) catheter (a flexible tube) and drain bag (below) is used for urine collection and measurement. The catheter, inserted and not changed for weeks, becomes a conduit to allow bacteria to migrate to the bladder and cause infections. The less time with an "indwelling" catheter the better, so ask when the Foley was first inserted, how often it is changed and if and when it can be removed and discontinued while your loved one is still in the hospital. The date it was first inserted and the planned removal date should be in the chart.

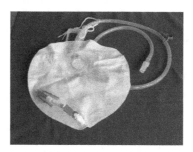

Foley

Keep it clean
Make sure the drain bag, which hangs on the bed frame, does not lie on or even touch the floor. If it touches the floor, ask the nurse to either change the bag or thoroughly wipe the bag with a disinfectant. No matter what, the bag should be wiped with a disinfectant as often as possible. Make sure nurses and caregivers wash their hands or put on gloves before touching the Foley and catheter.

Get it removed as soon as allowed
As the discharge date approaches, ask when the Foley system will be removed. If your loved one has a chronic (long-term) problem with the bladder fully emptying, residual urine will

create a higher risk of chronic bladder infection, so ask the doctor about removing residual urine from the bladder using "intermittent catheterizing" at home (temporary placement of a sterile catheter to remove urine from the body) to reduce the frequency of bladder infection. For more tips on infection prevention and more information about intermittent catheterizing, see page 173.

Keep track of Medicare and insurance stay limits.

Ask the hospital discharge coordinator how many days your loved one has left within covered hospital stay limits. This person directs the daily operation of record processing to ensure discharge records are properly received, organized and forwarded to the appropriate physician for completion.

For more information on Medicare hospital stay coverage, see Medicare And You, 2010 (web pdf page 120):

http://www.medicare.gov/Publications/Pubs/pdf/10050.pdf

Repeat Hospital Stays And Medicare Limits

How long may I stay in a hospital under Medicare?

If it were one long uninterrupted stay, it would be 60 + 30 + 60 = 150 total days covered. When you are admitted to the hospital, you start using the first 60 days as "full" paid days (no per day co-pay), after the deductible. The next 30 days (61-90) are covered, but you will pay a per day co-pay. At day 91, you will start using the last 60 days (91-150) covered as "lifetime reserve" days and you will pay a higher per day co-pay.

How much is the deductible and the co-pay?

The hospital deductible for 2010 is $1,100 per benefit period. There is no daily co-pay during the first 60 days. The co-pay during days 61-90 is $275 per day and the co-pay for days 91-150 is $550 per day. Source: Medicare And You, 2010 (web pdf page 120).

http://www.medicare.gov/Publications/Pubs/pdf/10050.pdf

What if my stay is less than the maximum allowed (150 days), but I have to come back to the hospital for another stay?

If you are discharged from a hospital stay and do not return for at least 60 calendar days, the first 90 days (60 full and 30 co-pay) will be replenished. Upon return, you will be in a new benefit period and start over at day one by paying the hospital deductible again.

If you are readmitted sooner than 60 days, you will be in the same benefit period, so all days (full and co-pay) used during the last stay still count (are not replenished) and the hospital deductible paid for the previous stay will still apply. But, you will be much closer to using days 61-90 (with a per day co-pay) and to days 91-150 (with a higher per day co-pay) lifetime reserve days.

What are lifetime reserve days?

If you were to stay 90 days straight or have many stays without a 60 calendar day break between any of them, you would remain in the same benefit period, eventually reaching day 91, when you would start using up your 60 lifetime reserve days. Every lifetime reserve day used is gone forever. They are not replenished even after a 60 calendar day interval away from the hospital.

What if I have no full, co-pay or lifetime reserve days left and I go back to the hospital before 60 calendar days have passed?

If you have used all your covered days and can't stay away for 60 calendar days, you'll have no Medicare coverage when you return to the hospital. If you spend 60 days away, you start a new benefit period, so the first 90 days would be replenished and you would again pay the hospital deductible.

Does Medicare cover my loved one alone in a hospital room?

If your loved one needs to be "in isolation" because of an antibiotic resistant infection and if no single occupancy room is available, Medicare will cover your loved one alone in a double occupancy hospital room until a single room is available.

Returning To The Hospital

What non-emergency procedures require a trip to the hospital?

There are many reasons to briefly re-visit the hospital after going home, including chemotherapy (cancer treatment), dialysis (a treatment to replace kidney function), replacing a feeding tube and blood transfusions.

What is the frequency of feeding tube replacement?

Expect to return every six to nine months to have the feeding tube replaced (page 189). It is not high risk, so after a brief time of post-operative monitoring, your loved one should be able to go home the same day.

What about the tube feeding formula if my loved one must return and be admitted to the hospital for an overnight or longer stay?

If your loved one is tube fed, the formula or mix of formulas used at home has been working well if there has been no constipation or diarrhea. The hospital may not use the same formula (or it may be out of stock), which may cause digestive problems. Take a supply of formula to the hospital and ask the nurses to use it. Post a notice in the room and put the containers where they can be seen.

What about an occasional blood transfusion?

The potential of serious complications requires it to be done at the hospital. The procedure itself is not complicated, but any complication during a transfusion is very serious.

Chapter 2

Before Leaving The Hospital:
Questions To Ask Doctors And Nurses

This chapter explains what to ask healthcare professionals well before your loved one is discharged from the hospital, so you can become better informed about your loved one's ongoing home healthcare and can make proper arrangements ahead of time for home healthcare goods and services. Topics include:

Your becoming familiar in the use of medical devices and daily bedside tasks for continued healthcare at home

Requesting exit examinations by doctors and nurses regarding your loved one's medical conditions

The safe resumption of medicines at home

Monitoring and recording your loved one's health information at home

Free samples of hospital medical supplies to take home

Categories of providers of home healthcare medical goods and services

Bedside Care Training

What opinions and training should I seek before my loved one is discharged?

Bedside home healthcare devices
To acquire an understanding of home healthcare medical devices such as thermometers and blood pressure devices (pages 47-51), ask the nurses at the hospital for their opinions, recommendations and instruction.

Bedside home healthcare tasks
For medical conditions requiring care for your loved one at home, ask the nurses for training in the procedures and related equipment, which may include some of the ones mentioned below.

Oxygen equipment
Ask for training by a nurse and see Chapter 7, page 133.

Suctioning equipment
Ask for training by a nurse and see Chapter 8, page 149.

Nebulizer use
Ask for training by a nurse and see Chapter 9, page 171.

Intermittent catheterizing
Ask for training by a nurse and see Chapter 9, page 173.

Tube feeding
Ask for training by the nurse and see Chapter 10, page 179.

<u>Requesting Exit Examinations</u>

**What medical examinations and instruction should
I request before my loved one is discharged?**

Ask doctors and nurses to examine and review with you your
loved one's current and chronic medical issues. It will help
ensure your loved one will have appropriate attention before
leaving the hospital and will give you a starting point for
understanding care and follow up at home.

Eye exam and eye care
If there is a history of eye problems that need monitoring
and managed treatment, ask to have the eyes checked
by a doctor. A good example is Glaucoma, a condition of
excessively high pressure inside the eyeball. If there is dry
eye, ask about appropriate eye drops. Ask how to recognize
minor eye infections.

Mouth exam and mouth care
While at the hospital, ask nurses about mouth care and
recommended techniques, given your loved one's medical
condition. Issues include alternatives to tooth brushes and
what to observe when inspecting the mouth, teeth and gums.

Throat exam and tracheostomy care
If there is a tracheostomy (a surgically created hole in the
throat to allow air to pass), ask a doctor to remove the collar
system and check the condition of the opening, surrounding
tissue and the airway.

Before your loved one is discharged, you will need to receive
training from a nurse about daily tracheostomy care and
learn about issues particular to tracheostomy patients.

If your doctor recommends using a Passy-Muir valve (page 45) with the tracheostomy, ask a nurse to train you in its use and care.

Ear exam and cleaning
Request an ear examination and ask a nurse to show you how to effectively clean the ear canals and how often it should be done.

Skin exam and preventative care
Ask the doctor or nurse to examine your loved one for skin disorders, such as pressure ulcers and skin cancer. If they find anything needing further diagnosis and treatment, request a specialist to examine the skin areas in question.

Learn from the nurses how to recognize non-blanchable (reddened) skin areas. It may indicate a pre-pressure ulcer, so ask the nurse to show you how to relieve the pressure on the area and how to treat it.

Ask the nurses about a total skin care plan, which includes keeping your loved one clean at all times (so there is no urine or stool left against the skin), the use of lotions and creams as a skin barrier, how often and how to regularly turn your loved one to relieve pressure on susceptible skin areas and what to do if your training and diligence doesn't seem to prevent a skin problem from getting worse.

Feet exam and home care
If there are chronic foot problems or if the toenails need trimming, request a podiatrist. If your loved one is "homebound" (leaving the home requires considerable and taxing effort), Medicare may cover periodic podiatrist visits to the residence (page 177).

Dehydration and preventative care
This is a multifaceted problem. Ask about dehydration
risk and, given your loved one's age and condition, how
medication and feeding issues factor into dehydration. Learn
the warning sings of dehydration, like dark and concentrated
urine. For more information:

http://www.ascp.com/publications/tcp/1999/aug/prevention.shtml

Learn about pain issues
Ask the nurses and doctors what kind of pain your loved
one experiences, locations of recurring pain, predictability,
if pain is due to the medical condition, what to observe and
how to respond when your loved one seems to be in pain.

If there is an indication of pain, ask your loved one how
she feels. If your loved one can't speak, use a pain ruler to
discern the intensity of the pain and point to body areas to
locate it. To view a pain ruler, see page 51.

Pain can be underestimated, so be alert for wincing or
grimacing, a change in behavior or a subtle indicator, such
as the avoidance of certain activities, like passive or active
exercise (page 65).

Some pain may be normal or expected. Give your loved one
time off from physical therapy if she is having muscular pain
after working hard during previous exercise sessions. After
spending time in bed recovering without much movement,
temporary muscle pain from even mild exertion can affect
your loved one as it can any weekend warrior. For more
information, see this website and its many pain management
links:

If your loved one qualifies for the Medicare Home Health Benefit (page 58), a visiting nurse (page 60) may come to the residence to examine your loved one, perform many of these nursing tasks and may be able to refresh some of the training you requested at the hospital. They do not visit every day, so you will need to know how to perform daily medical care tasks specific to your loved one.

Hospital Discharge And Medicine Resumption At Home

What do we have to do to leave?

Discharge procedures are paperwork intensive, which includes the doctors on your loved one's case signing off. Once the doctor sets a discharge date, the discharge coordinator oversees the process, so ask her if there is anything you can do to keep things moving. If your loved one needs critical care transport home, discuss with the discharge coordinator the day and time of the transport.

What documents do I need to receive?

Get the discharge papers, which list procedures and medications given at the hospital during the stay up to and including the date of the discharge. They include regular medicines given, doses held (skipped per doctor's order), medicines permanently discontinued, new medicines started and anything extraordinary like anesthesia as part of a procedure. The documents provide continuity, so medicines and care can resume safely at home.

What should I ask the doctor about resuming medicines at home?

If your loved one had been under medical care at home and after discharge you will be resuming home healthcare, the hospital stay may have temporarily disrupted or changed the home medicine schedule. Referring to the discharge papers and your updated Medicines List (page 6), ask the doctor how, over the next 24 hours, to gradually ramp in ongoing and new medicines to safely get your loved one on schedule.

Ask the doctor to clarify which medicines should to be listed as discontinued, so you will no longer give them from your supply of medicines at home.

Medical Data Gathering and Tracking

What information should I track at home and what do I do with it?

Before your loved one leaves the hospital, ask the doctor what medical data you should be gathering and tracking at home and how often. Information may include monitoring and recording vital signs (e.g. heart rate, blood pressure) and additional medical data (e.g. blood sugar levels, urine production).

Ask a nurse at the hospital to teach you the techniques to obtain the data and to recommend the home care bedside equipment you should obtain. You can use a pulse oximeter (page 47) for the blood oxygen level and to determine the heart rate, but ask also how to feel and time the pulse in case the oximeter doesn't give an accurate heart rate. You will need a blood pressure device (page 49) for blood pressure readings. For body temperature readings, you will need a thermometer (page 47).

Ask the doctor how often you should call to report the status of your loved one and what changes in data or your loved one's appearance should prompt a call. Ask about normal data ranges and what to expect, given the age and condition of your loved one.

In addition to the medical information you will record at home, it is helpful to start a journal of each day's home healthcare issues, upcoming events and extra information relevant to your loved one's ongoing care. The creation and usefulness of a journal are further explained on page 119.

Vital signs record
Ask a nurse to train you to take vital signs, so you can maintain a record (below) at intervals recommended by the doctor. Use a dedicated notebook, so you will have an unbroken series of data columns to be able to see trends. Keep it by the bed to make entries and for quick reference.

Date & Time	Heart Rate (/Min.)	Blood Press.	Temp. (F.)	Breaths (/Min.)	Blood Oxygen%
1/1/2010					
7 A.M.	60	120/80	98.6	16	100
11 A.M.	65	124/82	98.8	19	98

Vital levels fluctuate with circumstance, so make a brief note next to each set of readings, for example if taken while asleep, awake, sitting up or during or soon after exercise. Note when antibiotics or other medicines like blood pressure management medicines are started, so when you scan a column of changes over time, you can easily spot positive or negative trends and identify possible causes. If you need to call the doctor, the current readings and the trends are very important. The more disciplined information you make available to a doctor, the more help you are. If you have to

38

take your loved one to the ER, bring the notebook.

Are there specific things to monitor and record if my loved one is being tube fed?

If your loved one is being tube fed, ask if you should list the daily (every 24 hours) volume of liquid formula consumed. If water can only be given through the feeding tube, ask if you should record the daily water amount as well. Ask about keeping track of daily urine output and bowel movements. A record of the daily volume of "liquids in" and "liquids out" helps the doctor with his assessments.

Why should I care about measuring urine output?

The doctor can use an accurate measure of urine output to help assess your loved one's medical condition, for example hydration and dehydration. If you keep track of how much fluid goes in (as water, other liquids and tube feeding formula) and out (as urine) each day, you can be a great help to the doctor. Record this information in your journal.

Should I and how do I keep track of bowel movements?

If your loved one doesn't have a regular and formed stool, ask the doctor if you should chart bowel movement to estimate the fluid loss from diarrhea and record trends to report to the doctor. Ask a nurse to show you how.

You can help the doctor, because your chart will show when a new pattern started and if it's getting better or worse. If the doctor responds with an order, charting can provide feedback to let the doctor know how well it worked. Charting can keep the tube feeding formula osmolality mixture on target (page 182) to avoid constipation and diarrhea.

<u>Standard Information Gathering</u>

What general information should I gather at home?

The daily summary and doctor's order record can be entered in the daily journal (page 119). Ask the nurses at the hospital to show you how they record the information.

Daily summary
Ask a nurse about what to include, so at the end of each day, you can summarize healthcare events and medical conversations. This information should be recorded in your journal. The daily summary may be helpful to doctors and nurses in assessing your loved one's condition, because it provides context to raw data like the vital signs record (page 38).

Doctor's orders record
When taking a doctor's order (treatment or medication instructions) over the phone, write the doctor's name, the order and the date and time the order was received. If a nurse calls on behalf of the doctor to relay the order, list her name as well.

After you write a phone order, look at your written text and read it back to the doctor or nurse, so she can tell if you fully understood the order and wrote it down clearly. This extra step will help ensure a visiting nurse or anyone else reading the order will interpret it as intended.

If there are others helping out with caregiving, make a copy of the order and post it to be seen and read. Each reader should initial and date the posted copy. As you may have done at the hospital, post notices of allergies above the bed.

The following records and lists were discussed in Chapter 1 and are mentioned again to emphasize their importance as part of home healthcare.

Medicine Chart
Fill out a new chart (Appendix 3) every day with doctor's orders of prescription medicines, over the counter (OTC) medicines and supplements, how they are to be given and the dosages. Record the dates and times of each dose given, any doses skipped per doctor order and anything discontinued, including the final dose of an antibiotic.

Keep updating these records
Regularly update the Medical History, the Medicines List and the Side Effects/Allergies List (pages 5-6).

The following lists will help you organize your interaction with doctors and hospitals.

Doctor Information List
At the hospital, you gathered your loved one's doctors' and nurses' contact information (Appendix 1) . As more health professionals become involved, add them to the list.

Home Healthcare Contact Information List
Update this list (Appendix 2) of preferred medical supply companies, visiting nurse agencies and nurses as well as mobile X-ray (page 54) technicians. Include notes about terminated or rejected persons or companies.

<u>Free Samples Of Medical Disposables</u>

Are there any "freebies" (free samples) to start us off with an initial supply of home healthcare medical disposables?

During the hospital stay, make notes of the disposables and other items being used in the hospital your loved one will also need at home. For an initial home healthcare supply, ask a nurse to help you identify those items and to give you some of each during the discharge process.

After you use up your initial supply of "free samples", Medicare and insurance may not cover re-supplying all of them. However, if your loved one qualifies for the Medicare Home Health Benefit (page 58), visiting nurses are supposed to bring to the residence all covered equipment and disposables related to the completion of their tasks.

Here are some examples of common disposable medical supplies:

Alcohol prep pads
Used to disinfect skin surfaces, they can also be used to clean the earpieces of a stethoscope before each use to prevent an ear infection.

Disposable surgical masks
Get a box of masks, so when you aren't feeling well, you can still be at the bedside at home. Masks need to be regularly changed and disposed of, because they will become ineffective after becoming moist from your breath.

Disposable gloves
Get a box of disposable gloves. Some people are allergic to

latex, so get a box of non-latex gloves as well. Try them on to make sure they fit.

Wound dressing creams
Ask the nurses what creams were used at the hospital and request a couple of extra tubes until you can get more from your pharmacy.

Paper thermometers
Request a week's supply. Your pharmacy should carry them (page 47) as well.

60 cc catheter tip syringes
If your loved one is being fed through a tube to the stomach or small intestine, ask a nurse to get you a few of these syringes (below) to give medicine and water via the tube and to clear tube clogs. Have the nurse train you in these procedures (pages 185-188).

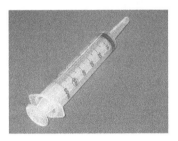

60 cc Catheter Tip Syringe

Tracheostomy canulas
The canula (below) is a removable inner airway tube, which inserts and locks into a tracheostomy (a surgically created hole in the throat to allow air to pass) tube collar system.

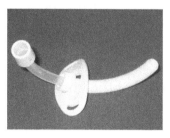 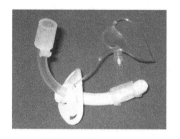

Cuffless Tube System   Cuffed Tube System
(canula partially removed)   (canula partially removed)

Cuffed canulas (above right) are for ventilator (a machine used to assist breathing) patients. Ask the doctor to recommend the right tube collar system and canula.

A reusable canula is cleaned daily and replaced as directed. A disposable canula doesn't need to be cleaned, because it is replaced with a new one each day. If you don't want to clean the canula every day, ask the doctor to order a disposable canula tracheostomy tube system.

Ask the nurse for some spare canulas that fit your loved one's collar system. Tube systems and canulas are prescription items, so you cannot order them direct. Ask your pharmacy to order them. Medicare may cover canulas and their tube systems. Our pharmacy ordered from Covidien:

http://www.nellcor.com/prod/Product.aspx?S1=AIR&S2=TTA&id=144

Five designations of a tracheostomy tube:

Brand
Product model
Type   (cuffed or cuffless)
Size number   (diameter of opening: 4, 6...)
Reusable or disposable

Passy-Muir valve
This air valve (below) fits like a cap on the exposed end of the tracheostomy tube canula and is used to block outgoing air pressure from the opening, so tracheostomy patients can be heard when they speak. The valve must be completely dry to operate properly. Request two valves, so a dry one is always ready and can be used if the other is still drying after being cleaned. They last a long time, but if you need replacements, see this website for ordering information and Medicare reimbursement codes.

http://www.passy-muir.com/products/pmvs/order-patient.aspx

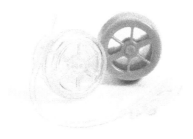

Passy-Muir Valves

Ask a nurse to train you in the care and use of Passy-Muir valves. Don't use them unless you are professionally trained first.

Y port tube feeding adapter
If your loved one has tube feeding (Chapter 10), request spare adapters. On the side of the adapter, you can see a small side port. This port is used to infuse medicines without the need to interrupt the feeding pump. For some added benefits of using an adapter, see page 192.

An adapter (below) lasts about six months. If your loved

one qualifies for the Medicare Home Health Benefit (page 58), you may be able to get free replacements from visiting nurses. If not, you can buy adapters from Internet vendors with possible Medicare coverage (see website below and Appendix 5).

http://www.apria.com/branch_locator1/1,3577,496-California,00.html

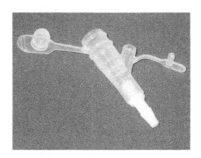

Y Port Tube Feeding Adapter

We don't qualify for the Home Health Benefit. Can we get durable medical equipment related disposables covered at home?

Medicare covers durable medical equipment (DME) (Chapter 4) and related disposables under a different provision from the Home Health Benefit.

Disposable oxygen masks and tubes may be covered with oxygen bottles and oxygen concentrators (Chapter 7); disposable air-filters and catch jars may be covered with home suction machines (Chapter 8); tube feeding formulas and bags may be covered with tube feeding pumps (Chapter 10).

Home Healthcare Bedside Devices

What types of bedside home healthcare devices should I ask the doctor and nurse about?

Thermometer types
The paper type (below left) can be hard to read, but is useful if your loved one won't "open wide" or lift the tongue. The digital one (below right) needs a hearing aid sized battery and beeps when the reading in Celsius (C.) or Fahrenheit (F.) is ready. It has a tiny battery, like one used in a hearing aid, but will not be accurate if the battery is low. Oral and rectal mercury thermometers (not shown) are inexpensive and accurate, but can they break and leak toxic mercury.

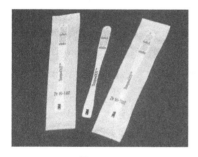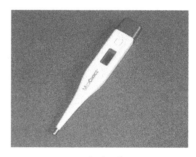

Paper   Digital

Pulse oximeter use
A pulse oximeter is used if a patient's blood oxygenation is unstable as in emergencies and intensive care or whenever there is a need to assess a patient's oxygenation or to determine the effectiveness of the supplemental oxygen.

A finger pulse oximeter (below) is suitable at home. It opens like a clothespin on the end of the finger and displays a numerical reading of the heart rate and the oxygen saturation level of arterial blood. Normal readings are 95-

100%, but the doctor will decide what is acceptable.

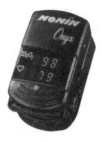

Finger Pulse Oximeter
(Image courtesy of Nonin Medical, Inc.)

A finger pulse oximeter may not display an accurate heart rate or blood oxygen level reading if the fingertip is too cold or the fingernail has nail polish or the pulse oximeter batteries are low. Usually, the device requires AAA size batteries. Other oximeter types use wired sensors with adhesive tape to attach to a finger, toe or earlobe.

Medicare doesn't cover these devices and prices vary, so shop around. Search the Internet using the keywords: pulse oximeter.

Stethoscope
Ask the doctor if a stethoscope is needed, for example, to determine the heart rate, check the lungs for congestion or take blood pressure readings.

If you are going to use a stethoscope, get trained by a nurse and before use, wipe the earpieces with an alcohol prep pad to prevent ear infection.

Using a stethoscope at home without adequate training may confuse more than clarify the situation. If you are not trained how and where to listen and if you don't have much experience to interpret what you hear, you won't be able to provide the doctor with useful information over the phone.

To avoid using a stethoscope, ask the doctor about using a pulse oximeter to measure the heart rate as part of the vital signs record (page 38). To take blood pressure readings, ask about using a digital blood pressure device instead of the manual type, which needs a stethoscope.

Manual blood pressure device
The traditional analog type has an air bulb to manually pump the arm cuff with air. It is aneroid (mercury-free) if it uses a dial gauge instead of a column of mercury to indicate the blood pressure.

Blood pressure is the force exerted by the blood against the walls of the arteries. A higher (systolic) number measures the force while the heart pumps blood and a lower (diastolic) number measures the force while the heart rests between beats. For more information about blood pressure numbers and what they mean:

http://www.americanheart.org/presenter.jhtml?identifier=4473

Digital blood pressure device
The battery powered digital type is easier to operate, because you don't need to listen to the blood flow with a stethoscope as with a manual one. The digital device displays a large font numerical readout and most models remember past readings for later display. It may give an error message if the arm cuff isn't on correctly or the batteries (usually, C size) are low. It may lose accuracy from changes in body position or due to an irregular heart rate during the use of the device.

If you need to take blood pressure readings, you can get either type of device from a discount pharmacy or the Internet. Ask the doctor what is normal blood pressure for your loved one and ask a nurse to train you to use the device.

Remote pacemaker testing
If your loved one has a pacemaker, ask the hospital to provide portable pacemaker testing equipment and instruction to test the pacemaker over the home phone line, so your loved one won't have to leave home. Ask the doctor how often the test needs to be conducted.

Glucometer kit
This device tests the blood glucose level (blood sugar). The kit should come with a supply of lancets (disposable needles to insert into the glucometer). When the glucometer is pressed against the fingertip, the short lancet needle snaps against the skin to create a drop of blood. The blood is absorbed by the test strip, which is then inserted into the glucometer.

If the doctor wants the blood sugar level monitored at home, you'll need a prescription specifying the number of tests per day to indicate how many lancets and test strips you will use in each 30-day period. You can get monthly supplies from your pharmacy and, if your loved one has Medicare, ask the pharmacy to submit for reimbursement. Ask a nurse to train you to use the glucometer.

Pain ruler
A pain ruler is a nonverbal way of finding out how much your loved one hurts. Your loved one (or you) points to a facial expression of pain on the pain intensity scale (below top) and you can match the selection with a pain description on the other side (below bottom). Read it aloud to your loved

one to confirm the intensity level, while pointing to and identifying the area of pain. For more information about pain management, see page 35.

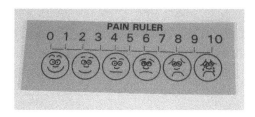

Pain Ruler (front)

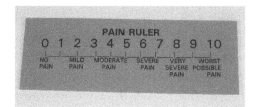

Pain Ruler (back)

Providers Of Home Healthcare Equipment, Services And Supplies

Who provides home healthcare medical goods and services?

Hospital based departments and private companies specialize in home healthcare medical goods and services. Some services, such as visiting nurses and specialty pharmacy prescriptions may be available from hospitals, independent companies and nurse registries, but if a service like mobile X-rays is not offered by the hospital, you will have to select an independent company. Medicare and insurance coverage are not dependent on providers being hospital based, but make sure they "accept assignment"

(Medicare allowed prices).

What about referrals to home healthcare companies?

Be extremely careful about hospital staff referrals to private home healthcare companies. A hospital employee could have an undisclosed family or business relationship. An unreasonable, unethical company could be an impediment to your loved one's care. If a company is rigid and confrontational, it will add to your stress level.

Allow enough time before the discharge date to do an independent check of all referrals. Start at least two weeks prior to the planned discharge date and if you can, investigate each company by speaking with the owners, managers and customers. Ask doctors for recommendations.

Here are some home healthcare providers and tips:

Specialty Pharmacies

What are specialty pharmacies?

This is not the same as a retail drug store. Also known as compounding pharmacies, specialty pharmacies pre-mix medicines for intravenous (IV), injected and inhaled methods. Your hospital may have a home healthcare specialty pharmacy, but if not, drugstore chains like Walgreens own and operate specialty pharmacies.

Check out recommended specialty pharmacies and have one selected before your loved one is discharged. If you make a choice without asking questions, you may be disappointed on every question I have listed below. Ask specialty pharmacies these questions, so you can choose one to treat you fairly.

Does the specialty pharmacy require your loved one to pay all or part of the Medicare allowed amount at delivery?

No, they should be willing to bill Medicare and insurance first.

Is there a delivery charge?

No, there shouldn't be.

On weekends and holidays, do they charge extra to "open up" the specialty pharmacy?

They should never charge to open the pharmacy.

Will they re-do the prescription at no charge if it is filled incorrectly, because of a miscommunication between the prescribing doctor and the specialty pharmacy?

Yes, they should be willing to correct a mistake.

If someone at home drops or spills a dose so it's not usable, will they provide a free replacement of the lost dose?

Some do, but don't expect this favor as routine.

Retail Drug Stores

What issues are there with retail drug store pharmacies?

Running out of medicines
Ask which medicines they are more likely to run out of if they don't have enough notice and how much notice they need.

Pain medications not in stock
Many pharmacies don't keep narcotic pain medications in stock and may need advance notice. Ask the doctor what she would prescribe and ask the pharmacy how much notice they need.

Hours of operation and delivery
Know their hours of operation and if they deliver during all business hours. Many pharmacies are open 24 hours, but some don't deliver on weekends, late evenings or at all.

Have an alternative
Consider having a relationship with more than one local pharmacy. If your usual pharmacy drops the ball, you can try the alternative.

Mobile X-ray And Diagnostic Testing Companies

My loved one can't leave home to get an X-ray.

X-rays are used to diagnose. A common X-ray order is a chest X-ray to see of there is a lung problem like pneumonia. Elderly persons with chronic (long-term) conditions are more susceptible to lung infections, especially if they are not able to get out of bed or walk on their own.

Mobile X-rays are usually available through a privately owned service. You can find them on the Internet using the keywords: mobile x-ray.

If the residence is in an area they cover, X-ray technicians with portable X-ray machines will come to the bedside to take X-rays and have them processed and sent to a radiologist for a written interpretation. The radiologist will fax the opinion to the doctor who ordered the X-rays.

If your loved one is "homebound" (leaving the home requires considerable and taxing effort), Medicare and insurance may cover mobile X-rays. Before you can confirm an appointment, the doctor must write a prescription specifying the reason for the X-rays and each area of the body to receive an X-ray. The doctor will fax the prescription to the X-ray company.

Be sure the company "accepts assignment" (Medicare allowed prices). Always ask if the X-ray company will first bill Medicare and insurance and not require your loved one to pay at the time of service. If a company insists on payment at the time of service, look for another company.

Are there additional mobile diagnostic services available?

Some mobile X-ray companies also perform these services:

Electrocardiograph (EKG), a machine to record electrical impulses generated in the heart, which produced as a paper graph, is used to diagnose heart function and conditions.

Ultrasound tests for vascular, venous, thyroid, heart and abdominal assessments.

Bone density scans of the patient's hand to determine overall bone density.

<u>Nurse Registries</u>

What about coverage for private nurses at home?

Home care private duty nursing (and caregiving) is available only through private agencies. They refer registered nurses (RNs), licensed vocational nurses (LVNs) and certified nurse assistants (CNAs). Medicare NEVER covers privately hired nursing services. Insurance might reimburse for a small number of private nurse hours logged per year.

We can't afford private duty nursing.

If your loved one has Medicare and qualifies for the Medicare Home Health Benefit, Medicare covers visiting nurses to the residence (explained in the next chapter).

Chapter 3

Before Leaving The Hospital:
Arranging Visiting Nurses And Therapists

If Medicare considers your loved one as "homebound" (leaving the home requires considerable and taxing effort), it means your loved one's medical condition may require special arrangements, for example a private ambulance service, to see a nurse or physical therapist. In this case, Medicare may cover nurses and physical, speech and occupational therapists to visit the residence.

This chapter explains the specific Medicare benefit covering nurse and therapist visits, how to qualify for the benefit, what visiting nurses do at the residence, how long and how often they visit and what is needed to have them continue to visit. How to arrange for regular recurring and extra visits is also discussed.

Visiting nurses are helpful in making sure your loved one receives the best care at home. They can reinforce some of the home care training you received at the hospital and they will give opinions about your loved one's current condition. These assessments will help the doctor maintain your loved one's health and promote improvement.

There are ideas to help your loved one recover strength at home. Examples of easy to use physical therapy equipment are provided, the use of which you can discuss with the therapist. Therapists can also help you plan and give appropriate exercise between the visits. Speech therapy, occupational therapy and other visiting services covered under the same benefit are explained.

Medicare Coverage For Nurse Visits

Can my loved one get visiting nurses paid by Medicare?

Yes, if your loved one qualifies for the Medicare Home Health Benefit. Therapists may be covered as well.

What is the Medicare Home Health Benefit?

It is a package of covered benefits paid by Medicare for those who need care at home. It covers skilled nursing visits to the residence by a registered nurse (RN) or a licensed vocational nurse (LVN) under the supervision of an RN. There are additional benefits under this provision, such as physical, speech and occupational therapist visits.

To receive Medicare coverage for any one of the benefits in this package, your loved one has to qualify for the Home Health Benefit by satisfying all conditions needed to qualify for all the benefits. To do this, the doctor must certify all of the following:

Homebound
Your loved one is "homebound" (leaving the home requires considerable and taxing effort).

Medical necessity
Your loved one has a (medically necessary) need for home healthcare and remains under a doctor's plan of care.

Skilled, part time and intermittent
Your loved one needs skilled physical or speech or occupational therapy services or skilled nursing on an "intermittent" (less than 7 days a week) or "part-time" (less than 8 hours a day) basis.

From an HHA
Your loved one receives the care from a Medicare approved Home Health Agency (HHA).

Additional Home Health Benefit Covered Services

What other services are also covered under this benefit?

The benefit also covers visits for evaluation, skilled therapy, home health aide services, medical social services and the use of medical equipment disposables directly related to a visiting nurse's bedside medical tasks.

Evaluation services
The benefit pays at least a portion of an evaluation visit by a skilled nurse or therapist.

Speech therapy (ST)
Therapists come to the residence to help your loved one regain and strengthen speech and language skills.

Occupational therapy (OT)
Therapists come to the residence to help your loved one practice at daily activities.

Home health aide services
A home health aide will visit to assist with personal care (e.g. bathing, using the toilet), but only if your loved one requires this in addition to requiring and being covered for a skilled (nursing or therapy) service. If your loved one needs only the services of a home health aide, she will not qualify for the Home Health Benefit and will not be covered for any services under the benefit, including this service.

Medical social services
Help or counseling with social or emotional concerns about the illness.

Medical supplies
Disposables, like dressings and catheters may be covered to enable the nurse to complete her tasks, but only if the visiting nurse brings them.

Skilled Nursing Visits

What is skilled nursing?

Depending on the medical complexity of the case and the tasks to be performed, either a registered nurse (RN) or a licensed vocational nurse (LVN) under the supervision of an RN may visit the residence to perform Medicare covered nursing services. Covered services are those that must be performed by a licensed nurse. Medicare does not cover medical tasks that can be safely performed by a non-medical person (including one's self) and tasks that do not have a legal requirement of direct supervision of a licensed nurse.

What do skilled nurses do during a visit?

A visiting nurse comes to the residence to perform tasks like drawing blood and taking samples to a laboratory. The nurse may check vital signs (e.g. blood pressure, heart rate), assess skin problems, look for edema (swelling), give medicines and injections, change wound dressings, clean the tracheostomy and canula (the incision in the front of the throat and the breathing tube), check intravenous (IV) lines and perform other medically necessary nursing tasks. Skilled nursing services also include training caregivers to perform bedside tasks and visits for the evaluation of your loved one's medical home care setting.

How long and how often are the visits?

A nurse visits only long enough to complete her tasks and visits must be "intermittent" or "part time" to be covered under the Medicare Home Health Benefit. The typical visit is one hour or less and the typical frequency is one to three times per week as directed by the doctor.

If your loved one doesn't need physical, speech or occupational therapy visits and needs only skilled nursing, then Medicare may cover either "intermittent" visits (less than 7 days a week) "as long as needed" or "continuous" (7 days a week) and "part time" daily (less than 8 hours a day) visits up to 2-3 weeks. "As long as needed" means visits under this benefit are covered by Medicare in 60-day cycles and must be re-certified (page 123) for the next 60 days at least every 60 days.

Medicare usually covers visits only if the "intermittent" (less than 7 days per week) and "part time" (less than 8 hours per day) visits do not exceed a total maximum of 28 hours per week. Depending on the medical need and on a case-by-case basis, the maximum may be allowed to increase to 35 hours per week.

If your loved one doesn't need any home nursing or needs it all the time without a foreseeable end date, your loved one cannot qualify for the skilled nursing part of the Home Health Care Benefit. Staying at the bedside after tasks are completed and watching a patient is considered private duty. Private-duty nursing is NEVER covered under any provision of Medicare.

What are important issues in scheduling nurse visits?

You want a standing order
For frequent and regular visits to perform the same tasks, the doctor can make it a standing (unending) order. A standing order is in effect until further notice, so the doctor doesn't have to re-request the same services every week. He needs to write the words "standing order" on the prescription.

With a standing order, nurses will be coming the same days and times each week, so it is more likely to be the same nurses each time. It's very important to maintain a consistency of nurses, because over time they will get to know your loved one and can notice if a condition has gotten better or worse since the previous visit.

Medicare visits still need to be re-certified every 60 days.

Some days are better than others
Mondays and Fridays are least preferable for visits, because visiting nurses take those days off more often. That means more visiting substitute nurses not as familiar with your loved one.

You prefer to be an early bird
The earlier in the day regular visits are scheduled, the earlier the laboratory report will be in the doctor's hands, the fewer calls you have to make in the afternoon to see if the doctor received the report and the earlier you can get an opinion from the doctor. If there is a mix up and a nurse doesn't show (page 120), you'll know it at an earlier hour and it will be much easier to get a nurse to come out while the day is still young.

Who provides visiting nurses?

Medicare covered intermittent and part time nurse visits to the residence are available from a hospital based home healthcare department approved by Medicare or from a private Medicare approved Home Health Agency (HHA).

How do I get the visiting nurses scheduled?

The doctor will request nurse visits on certain days of the week via a written order he will fax to a Medicare approved Home Health Agency (HHA), which may be the hospital home healthcare nursing department or an independent nurse registry. Once the HHA determines the care is covered, they will schedule visits.

What is required on a faxed visiting nurse order?

Ask the agency and go over the following list:

- Patient name
- Doctor name
- Doctor's signature or stamp
- Date of the order
- Date of the requested visit (or)
- Date of the first visit of a standing order
- Frequency of visits per week
- Preferred days of the week
- Procedure(s) ordered
- "Standing order" if visits are to continue indefinitely
- "STAT" for an extra visit on short notice

Nurse visitation orders are called "referrals" by visiting nurse agencies.

What can I do to head off problems with a faxed order?

Ask the doctor's office to fax you a copy of the visiting nurse order. Examine it to make sure the order information required by the agency is complete and accurate. If an order has the wrong date requested or is lacking necessary information, an agency usually won't schedule the visit and may not call the doctor to inform him the order has a problem.

Once you have checked the order, call the nursing agency to ask if they received their copy. If they haven't, you can fax your copy to them and not bother the doctor's office. Confirm they got the fax and write the name of the person with whom you spoke on the back of your copy.

Physical Therapy Visits To The Home

What rehabilitation resources are available?

If your loved one is well enough to leave home, Medicare covered physical, speech and occupational therapy sessions can be given as directed at a Medicare approved therapy center.

My loved one has not recovered well enough to leave home to go to a physical therapist.

If your loved one is considered "homebound" (leaving the home requires considerable and taxing effort), she has met one of the conditions, all of which must be met, to qualify for the Medicare Home Health Benefit (page 58), which covers visiting therapists as well as visiting nurses.

How do we get covered visiting therapists to come to our home?

Before your loved one leaves the hospital, ask the doctor to write an order stating your loved one is "homebound" (leaving the home requires considerable and taxing effort) and home physical therapy is needed. The doctor must fax the order to a Medicare approved Home Health Agency (HHA), which schedules the visits.

Getting Therapy Organized

What should I ask the physical therapist regarding appropriate exercises?

Ask a physical therapist to demonstrate and draw diagrams of appropriate passive (range of motion) and active exercises, so you will know how to exercise your loved one at home. Ask the doctor and nurse to review the suggested exercises to make sure you won't "over do it" and cause exhaustion, injury or skin pressure problems.

If you take your loved one to a physical therapy center or have a visiting physical therapist coming to the residence, ask the therapist to recommend and regularly re-evaluate the exercises you may use at home between professional sessions.

What is passive and active exercise?

Passive exercise is performed when a patient is unable to exercise on his own. It involves the manual manipulation of parts of the body to extend the range of motion and reduce muscle atrophy (loss of mass and strength due to lack of use). Passive exercise is taking place when the exercise is for avoiding pain and exertion while maintaining and extending the range of motion for areas like the shoulders.

Active exercise is done with your loved one's participation by actively flexing muscles to move parts of the body against some kind of resistance to build strength and endurance.

What specifically can my loved one and I do between professional physical therapy sessions?

Give passive (range of motion) exercise
Passively exercise your loved one as directed to conserve energy, manage fatigue and to increase the ranges of the exercised body parts to reach or stretch. Have the physical therapist list and demonstrate passive exercises, recommend their frequency and draw stick figure pictures of positions you can to refer to.

Provide active exercise
If your loved one can participate in active exercise, ask the physical therapist to list and describe appropriate active exercises, recommend their frequency and draw stick figure pictures of positions, so you can remember them.

Ask about exercise equipment
Some active exercises involve exercise equipment, so ask the therapist what equipment is appropriate for your loved one. After you purchase it, have the therapist train you for use between professional therapy sessions.

Affordable Exercise Equipment

What exercise equipment can be used at home?

The following physical therapy devices strengthen and

stretch. You can buy them from Internet vendors and although not expensive, they are not covered by Medicare or insurance.

Ask your physical therapist about these devices and after your doctor has approved exercises using them, ask the physical therapist to demonstrate the devices, draw stick figure position diagrams for your reference and to train you to use them to exercise your loved one between professional therapy sessions. Pictures follow their descriptions.

Pedaling machine
While sitting in a chair or a wheelchair, exercise the legs and ankles to increase endurance. When placed on a table or a wheelchair tray (page 105), it can be used to exercise the arms.

Quadriceps board
While in bed, exercise the quadriceps (front thigh muscles), which are essential for standing up and walking.

Ankle rocker
While sitting with the feet on the floor, stretch the ankles and related calve muscles to keep them flexible. Use it as directed to warm up before other exercises, like pedaling, standing or walking.

Exercise skate
Therapy may include swinging the leg (whose foot is strapped to the skate) out toward the edge of the bed and then bringing it back to the center. For this, you'll also need a 3-foot x 3-foot piece of ¼ inch thick plywood under the skate.

Therabands
Rolls of elastic bands can be cut into sections and tied in

loops for customized resistance exercises. They come in different colors, which indicate increasing levels of effort to stretch them.

Styrofoam roller
While in bed, it may be placed under parts of the body like the knees for raising the lower legs and under the thighs to try to raise the rear end off the bed.

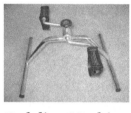
Pedaling Machine

Quadriceps Board

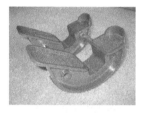
Ankle Rocker

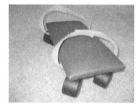
Exercise Skate

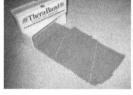
Theraband

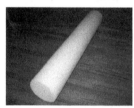
Styrofoam Roller

Additional Activities

What else can we do for exercise and stimulation?

Get a plastic beach ball
While having fun and feeling happy, your loved one may not realize how much he is exercising. You can toss the ball to him in the wheelchair or in bed and encourage him to throw it back under or over-handed. Eventually, he may lift the ball over his shoulders and head and throw it with both hands. You can play kickball by rolling it to him sitting in the

wheelchair (with the footrests removed), so he can kick it by swinging his legs. Playing ball stimulates vision, develops strength and increases coordination.

Get some party balloons
You can play balloon volleyball, reaching up and out to bat the balloon back and forth while your loved one is in bed or a wheelchair. When the balloon goes off course, it makes your loved one look for the ball, try to react to the randomness and reach out quickly to stay in the game. The unpredictability of the balloon path is very good for hand/ eye coordination. The larger, rounder, heavier balloons stay more on course than odd shaped ones.

Play games
Keep her mind busy. Play games, cards and listen to your loved one's favorite music (page 125).

Get your loved one out of the bedroom
After being cooped up in the hospital and then in the bedroom, getting out of the bedroom to other rooms will make your loved one feel like life is returning to normalcy. Going outside is even more stimulating and healing.

Call for visitors
Call your loved one's friends and let them know it's time for a visit. Sometimes, people are conflicted about coming over and need an invitation.

Preventing Foot Drop

What is foot drop?

Over time, without stretching or exercising, muscles and tendons of the ankles and feet can become weakened and stretched leading to a condition called foot drop. People with foot drop can't use the weakened ankle muscles to lift up their toes during strides. Unable to fully pick up their feet, the toes scrape the ground. Those who can walk, but have this condition have to change their way of walking to avoid tripping over their toes. If the person is too weak to walk at all and gets foot drop, it makes it nearly impossible to ever walk again.

How can I prevent it?

It is prevented with physical therapy for the lower legs, ankles and feet and keeping the feet from drooping forward during the night while sleeping. Multi podus boots are designed prevent foot drop by keeping the feet in a specific position while at rest.

What are multi podus boots?

Multi podus boots (below) keep feet in a standing position, so they can't droop and stretch out the ankle and foot muscles used to raise the toes while walking. Plastic tabs can extend perpendicularly from the boots to keep the feet and knees pointing upward.

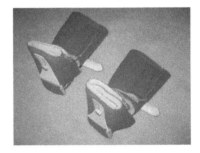

Multi Podus Boots

I can't afford the boots.

When your loved one is in bed, keep some pillows pushed between the feet and the foot of the bed. Ask a nurse or caregiver to show you. If you don't use the boots, keep an eye on the posture of the feet.

Chapter 4

Before Leaving The Hospital:
Arranging Home Healthcare
Durable Medical Equipment And Supplies

This chapter will help you plan and obtain your loved one's home healthcare durable medical equipment (DME) and supplies, such as a wheelchair, adjustable home healthcare bed, patient lift and sling, supplemental oxygen and tube feeding equipment.

The Medicare definition of covered durable medical equipment (DME) is reviewed along with the basics of coverage.

Home healthcare equipment companies are described to help you deal with them when selecting equipment. The equipment is detailed with tips for equipment upgrades and Medicare coverage.

If your loved one needs Medicare covered durable medical equipment and related disposable supplies at home, you must call a home healthcare company with a prescription several days in advance of planned delivery. Arrange it to be delivered and set up with training provided *well before your loved one leaves the hospital*, so you will have time to become familiar with the equipment and related supplies.

Durable Medical Equipment Defined By Medicare

What is durable medical equipment (DME)?

A durable good is a product that does not quickly wear out.

Medicare defines covered durable medical equipment (DME) as medical equipment that satisfies all four of these conditions:

Repeated use
It can withstand repeated use, so it could normally be rented and used by successive patients. Generally, this excludes disposable equipment and supplies used once or only a few times. However, disposables such as oxygen tubes and masks needed for covered oxygen equipment to function are covered as well.

Medical purpose
It is primarily and customarily used to serve a medical purpose. Your loved one must have a medical condition that the use of the DME, like a home healthcare bed, should improve or help prevent from getting worse.

Usefulness for illness or injury only
Generally, it is not useful in the absence of illness or injury. This excludes equipment designed solely to prevent injury, like bathroom grab bars.

Appropriateness for home healthcare
It is appropriate in a residence. This excludes exercise devices (pages 66-68) and physical therapy equipment like parallel bars, which are considered institutional.

The following websites provide more information regarding DME, which may be covered if specific medical conditions exist:

http://www.medicarerights.org

http://www.medicareinteractive.org

Home Healthcare Durable Medical Equipment Companies

Who provides home healthcare durable medical equipment and related disposable supplies?

Home healthcare companies supply durable medical equipment (DME) like home healthcare beds and wheelchairs as well as tube feeding pumps and formulas, oxygen equipment and bottles, bedside suction equipment and related disposables.

Where can I search for home healthcare companies and how should I select one?

You can find home healthcare companies that service your area on the Internet using the keywords: home healthcare. Some are local small businesses, usually situated near hospitals and some are larger chain locations servicing your area.

When considering which company to use, important points are: selection and availability of products and supplies, customer service handling your needs and concerns in a deliberate way, scheduling and being on time with deliveries and replacement equipment, providing training at home for delivered equipment and prompt billing of Medicare and insurance.

I am being told I must use the same home healthcare company for all home healthcare equipment needs.

That's not correct. You can use as many different companies as you like. However, it is simpler the fewer you use.

Home Healthcare Company Tips

The company is requesting a credit card.

Even if you have Medicare and insurance, some companies will start out requiring a credit card for co-pays or in case coverage is denied. Tell their billing office the card is not to be used for routine bills; they must bill only via periodic statements. Once you establish a good payment history, ask them to shred your card information.

Can I get a monthly statement?

Some companies send quarterly (every three months) statements. If you want a statement each month, make it a special request with their billing department.

The home healthcare company representative is going too fast with so much information.

The home healthcare company will send a representative to the hospital or your loved one's residence to help you understand and obtain home healthcare equipment and supplies. At the hospital, the meeting with the representative is usually close to the discharge date. This is a new area, so slow it down and discuss each piece of equipment, ask about options and write down the answers. You are not required to make snap decisions or sign contracts, so take your time and know you can always change your mind.

I want to verify coverage information and options regarding the equipment our representative discussed with us.

If something doesn't sound accurate or if the representative seems vague, is not an effective communicator or is not as knowledgeable as you expected, you may want a second opinion. Call customer service and ask about the same items to make sure your understanding is correct.

What could a follow up phone call reveal?

The representative could be misinformed or forget to mention options. If you are told something is not covered, the item might be covered if the doctor fills out medical necessity forms. Or, there might be a less expensive covered version of the denied equipment. A phone call to another representative from the same company or a competitor can reveal options and even save money.

What commitments should I get from the representative?

He will submit claims on your behalf
If the home healthcare company is supplying you with Medicare covered equipment costing less than $150 like a walker or commode or the equipment is made to order, you will have to buy it, but the home healthcare company must submit a claim to Medicare on your behalf (page 80). Get assurance from the company representative the claims will be submitted. To help ensure he follows through, let him know you regularly review your quarterly Medicare statement (MSN).

He will inquire about coverage for an air mattress system (LAL) or an air mattress pad (APP)
If your loved one is Medicare covered for a home healthcare bed and you are concerned with the healing or prevention of bedsores, ask about a continuous low air loss mattress (LAL) (page 87) or an alternating pressure pad (APP) (page 89).

The bed comes with a foam mattress, but Medicare will not cover the more expensive LAL unless there are bedsores. If there are none, ask about the less expensive APP. An APP lies on top of the foam mattress and depending on the needs and condition of your loved one, may be Medicare covered to prevent bedsores.

He will provide new equipment
You will not do business with him unless he provides new or "like new" equipment. As you will see (page 84), this is important.

Equipment Coverage Basics

What are the ways Medicare pays for DME?

Depending on the classification of the equipment and the needs and condition of your loved one, here are four ways Medicare may cover an item:

Buy it outright
The equipment, for example a scooter or motorized wheelchair, then belongs to your loved one.

Rent it continuously
The rent continues until the equipment is no longer needed.

Consider the equipment as capped rental, rent it for a set period of time and then give it to your loved one
The equipment is rented for 13 months (except capped rental oxygen equipment) and then is given to your loved one. Medicare pays 80% of the allowed monthly rent for 13 continuous (without a break) months and at month 14, transfers ownership.

For each of the first 13 months, your loved one pays (insurance may pay some of) the remaining 20% of the Medicare allowed monthly rent.

If your loved one doesn't need the capped rental equipment before the 13 continuous month period has elapsed, the supplier still owns it and will pick it up.

If your loved one purchases a capped rental item at the outset or before the 13 month capped rental period is complete, Medicare will not reimburse for it.

Once your loved one owns the equipment, Medicare will pay for a portion of the repairs, labor and replacement parts and for temporary loaner equipment during the time the equipment is away.

Capped rental oxygen equipment
It is rented for 36 (instead of 13) months, during which time Medicare covers all service, accessories and oxygen contents and at month 37, transfers ownership of the equipment to your loved one. If your loved one doesn't need the capped rental oxygen equipment (Chapter 7) for all 36 continuous months, the supplier will still own it and will pick it up.

After 36 months, Medicare will still cover replacement of oxygen accessories, monthly oxygen content and, at regular intervals, checking the oxygen equipment.

Is all Medicare covered DME classified as capped rental equipment?

Not all Medicare covered DME is considered capped rental equipment. Capped rental equipment includes manual and semi-electric home healthcare beds (not total electric), manual wheelchairs (not motorized), nebulizers, mattress overlays, manual patient lifts (not electric) and oxygen equipment.

What non-capped rental equipment will Medicare purchase?

Some expensive items, like motorized wheelchairs and scooters may be purchased and, if your loved one qualifies, Medicare may cover 80% of the allowed purchase amount. At the store, make sure they "accept assignment" (Medicare allowed prices) and find out what the allowed amount is.

Medicare Coverage For Durable Equipment Under $150

The home healthcare supply company says my loved one has to pay for low cost equipment like a walker or a commode. Doesn't Medicare cover this equipment?

Medicare requires your loved one to purchase covered home healthcare equipment if it is "made to order" (custom) or sells for less than $150. Your loved one would have to pay the home healthcare company in full at delivery, but the home healthcare company must bill Medicare on your loved one's behalf for 80% of the Medicare allowed amount. The difference (20%) is your loved one's out of pocket cost.

Submit the remaining 20% to insurance to see if they will reimburse you for a portion of it.

We bought these inexpensive items and were never reimbursed.

Unfortunately, a paid company has a diminished incentive to submit a claim. The home healthcare company representative should mention claims for these purchased items will be submitted to Medicare on your loved one's behalf. Bring it up when making the purchases and check your quarterly Medicare statements to be sure the claims were submitted for your reimbursement.

Lists Of Medicare Sometimes/Never Covered Equipment

What is sometimes covered and never covered?

Medicare doesn't cover DME for use primarily outside the home. If your loved one can walk around the inside of the home, Medicare will not cover a motorized scooter to get around outside. For a scooter to be covered, the doctor has to certify "limited mobility" inside and outside the home. Medicare will never cover equipment used for "convenience", such as stairway elevators, grab bars and toilet seats. Medicare never covers wheelchair ramps (purchased or built) or costs of home modifications for health care or to widen doors for wheelchair access. For more information about covered/denied durable medical equipment, see:

The Medicare National Coverage Determinations Manual (web pdf pages 87-97):

http://www.cms.hhs.gov/manuals/downloads/ncd103c1_Part4.pdf

Let's start with the bed. What are my options?

Manual bed
If your loved one's medical condition requires positioning of the body in ways not feasible with an ordinary bed such as to alleviate pain or elevate the head of the bed more than 30 degrees or for the use of traction equipment, Medicare may cover an adjustable, manually cranked bed (below left). Cranks (below right) raise and lower the head of the bed, the area under the knees and the bed elevation.

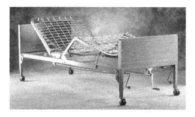   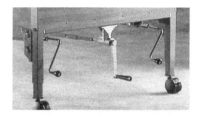

Manual Bed   Adjustment Cranks

Semi-electric bed
If your loved one needs frequent and/or immediate changes in body position, ask the doctor for a prescription to upgrade to a semi-electric bed (below left). It has an electric motor to independently raise and lower the head and knees, but still must be cranked to raise and lower the entire bed (below right). This is the Medicare coverage limit for a bed upgrade.

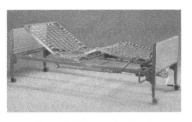

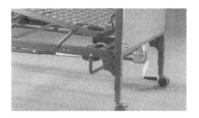

| Semi-Electric Bed | Elevation Crank |

Total electric bed
Medicare doesn't cover a total electric adjustable bed (below left). But, if you want to eliminate all cranking, you can obtain total electric bed by paying beyond what Medicare would pay for either the manual or semi-electric bed approved for your loved one. The total electric bed has a removable crank inserted at the foot of the bed (below right) in the event of power outages or motor failure. Tell everyone where the crank is stored.

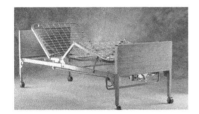

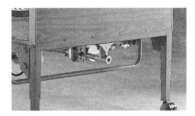

| Total Electric Bed | Removable Crank Socket |

If I pay extra for a bed upgrade, how does it work with the home healthcare company?

Manual and semi-electric beds are capped rental items
After 13 months, your loved one will own either the manual or semi-electric bed, depending on which one Medicare will cover. Depending on your loved one's needs, the prescription may get coverage for an upgrade to a semi-electric bed.

If you want to upgrade
To receive a total electric bed with Medicare contributing toward the cost, ask the supply company to deliver a total electric bed. Ask them to submit to Medicare for the bed type (manual or semi-electric) approved for your loved one and over the next 13 months, to apply those 13 Medicare monthly capped rental payments against the purchase price of the total electric bed.

After 13 months, the bed will be given to your loved one. This is after your loved one pays the difference between 13 Medicare payments plus 13 monthly co-pays already paid for the covered (manual or semi-electric) bed and the purchase price of the total electric bed.

If upgrading to a bed beyond what is covered, like a total electric bed, your loved one will pay the balance of the sale price to purchase the bed at the end of 13 months, so insist on a new bed.

When the bed was delivered, it wasn't new. If my loved one owns it after 13 months, it will be older than 13 months.

Correct. The equipment company is not obligated to start at month one with a brand new bed or, in general, any brand new capped rental equipment. They may have an inventory of used beds coming back from stints of less than 13 months and are sending them back out. If the supplier is replacing inventory, they might start with a brand new bed.

Capped rental equipment, like manual and semi-electric beds, must be rented for 13 continuous months for ownership to transfer (capped rental oxygen equipment is 36 months). If the bed is not at least "like new", tell them to replace it with a newer bed or you will go to another company for your all your medical equipment.

Bed Rails

What are bed rails and why are they necessary?

Made of tubular metal, rails are clamped onto the bed frame. Manually raising and locking the rails in the up position keeps your loved one from rolling out of bed. The down position is well below the top of the mattress for access to the bed. When ordering the bed, you can get two long rails (below left) or four short rails (below right).

Should I get two long bed rails or four short ones?

You might prefer the four short ones, because there is a gap between them at the center of the bed wide enough for your loved one to sit with legs over the bedside to exercise while holding onto the raised rails for support. Rails are included with the bed.

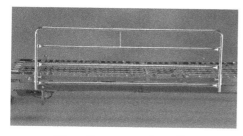
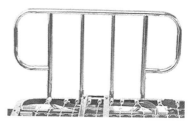

Two Long Bed Rails   Four Short Bed Rails

What are some hazards with bed rails?

Be very careful when releasing the rails for lowering. There is no dampening system, so once you pull the spring-loaded lock pin, the rail can drop like a stone. Make sure no fingers are in the way of the rails as they are lowered. Have a grip on the rail, so you can ease it down, but also make sure no toes are under the rails. If the bed elevation is low enough, the rail bottom can slam onto the floor and the toes.

Mattresses

What about the mattress?

Medicare will give your loved one a foam mattress with the (capped rental manual or semi-electric) bed frame. This basic mattress may be inadequate for your loved one's comfort or medical needs, especially if confined to a bed. Options are described below for immobile or bedridden patients, who are among the most susceptible to developing pressure sores.

What are pressure sores and who is most likely to get them?

Pressure sores are areas of damaged or broken skin. Sick people who sit or lie in one position too long can get them quite quickly. Without treatment, they can become deep wounds taking a very long time to heal. Pressure and shearing (friction against the skin surface) can damage the skin and increase the chance of a pressure sore. Areas of skin over bony parts of the body are most at risk. The most likely to get one are those who:

- Are very old or very young
- Are seriously ill, drowsy or unconscious
- Have had surgery
- Leak urine or feces
- Have a serious injury, such as a broken hip

- Are very overweight (obese)
- Don't eat or drink enough
- Have poor circulation, perhaps because of smoking
- Have had a pressure sore before
- Can't feel pain, which can happen if the spinal cord is injured or if diabetes has damaged the nerves

For more on the causes and prevention of pressure ulcers:

http://www.nursingassistanteducation.com/site/courses/eng/nae-ppu-eng.php

An appropriate bed and mattress is a good start, but you should also have a skin care plan, which includes the prevention and/or management of pressure ulcers, regular assessment by a nurse or doctor, appropriate turning and positioning, appropriate wound care, management of moisture and incontinence and nutritional assessment and intervention consistent with the overall plan of care.

I'm worried about bedsores. Isn't there something better than a foam mattress?

The devices described below are designed to help prevent and heal pressure sores on skin areas by distributing and changing the locations of pressure from body weight.

Continuous low air loss mattress (LAL)
If your loved one fits the Medicare coverage criteria, you may upgrade from the standard free foam mattress to an LAL, an air mattress with an air pump (below), which is used in many hospitals as part of a defense against bedsores. The large individual air cells have tiny pinholes to allow each cell to maintain constant air pressure while adjusting its shape to the weight and contour of the body. The air pump pressure

can be adjusted from soft to firm. While resting, your loved one may need medium support. To change a body position or if you want to sit your loved one up at the side of the bed, it is easier when the mattress pump is set to firm.

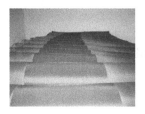 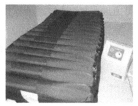 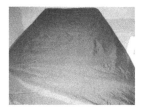

LAL Air Cells   LAL And Pump   LAL w/Cover

Coverage for an LAL
Medicare will not cover a low air loss mattress unless your loved one already has multiple Stage II bedsores (pressure ulcers) on the trunk and/or pelvis and then may do so only after Medicare specified ulcer treatment/prevention protocols have been tried. If the medical profile meets all the requirements and you have an appropriate prescription from the doctor, Medicare may cover this system. If you buy one to help prevent ulcers, Medicare will not consider coverage.

LAL air pump filter cleaning
If the air filter is dirty, the air pump (below left and center) will not be able to supply enough pressure to create the level of firmness desired. Slide the filter out of its slot (below right), squeeze it a few times under running water and slide it back in.

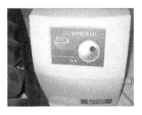 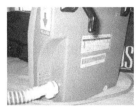 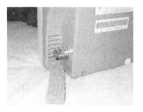

| LAL Air Pump | Reverse View | Foam Air Filter |

I can't get coverage for a continuous low air loss mattress (LAL) and I can't afford to buy one.

Alternating pressure pad (APP)
To help prevent bedsores with a Medicare covered mattress overlay, look into an APP (below left). Like a continuous low air loss system (LAL), it uses an air pump to fill its air cells.

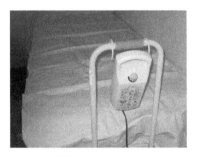 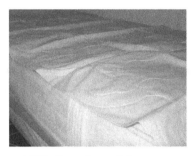

| APP And Pump | APP Overlays Mattress |

The difference between an APP and an LAL
An APP is a mattress pad designed to lie on top of a mattress (above right). An LAL is an air mattress. Both types help to distribute the pressure from body weight, so areas of skin are relieved before the pressure can begin to create problems.

An APP has many closed (no pinholes) small cells, which are automatically and alternatively inflated and deflated by an air pump. An LAL has larger and fewer open (pin-holed) cells with constant pressure from an air pump to adapt to body weight and shape. Some LAL systems can also automatically alternate pressure across their cells (like an APP).

If you consider an APP or an LAL, ask how to clean the air pump filter.

Medicare coverage for an APP
Your loved one must be completely immobile or have limited mobility with at least one additional condition: impaired nutritional status, incontinence, altered sensory perception or compromised circulatory status.

Wedge Pillow

What is a wedge pillow and how can it help?

This is a large wedge shaped piece of foam with a removable machine washable cloth cover. Even with a home healthcare bed to elevate the upper body and a great air mattress system, consider getting a wedge pillow. Spending time in bed with the head and upper body elevated can cause the back to be slightly bent and the shoulders turned inward toward the chest.

During waking hours, place the wedge pillow behind the elevated upper body and split the desired head elevation of the bed with the extra elevation of the wedge pillow to recline against a flatter and firmer surface than the mattress alone would provide. Your loved one's back will be straighter, the shoulders further back and the chest more expanded. This allows for deeper breathing and counteracts the shortening of chest muscles that may result from long periods in bed.

There are many shaped pillows available for your loved one's comfort and medical needs, so ask the doctor which is the most appropriate.

The pillow shown below is called a Duro-Med Bed Wedge (24 x 24 x 12 inches), product code: DUR-8028B. You can find vendors on the Internet with this keyword description. You must buy new, they are not returnable due to hygiene issues, are not covered by Medicare or insurance, but they are inexpensive, about $30.

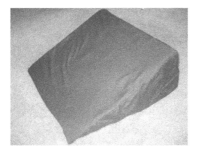
Wedge Pillow

Patient Lifts

My loved one can't stand up, so how do we move her?

Part of the home healthcare process may be routinely transferring your loved one to and from a bed, wheelchair and portable commode.

The method of transfer
The transferring method you should use will depend on your loved one's medical condition, strength, coordination, mental and neurological status, ability to move and/or stand and any pain experienced during or from a particular transfer method. It is also a function of your strength,

confidence and ability to transfer your loved one safely. Ask nurses and therapists to recommend the best transfer method for you and your loved one and to train you and anyone assisting you.

When a lift makes sense
Medicare may cover a manually operated patient lift (below left) if a transfer requires the assistance of more than one person and if, without the use of a lift, your loved one would be confined to a bed. If you have studied the user manual and have been trained by a professional and demonstrated through practice a proficiency with a lift and sling (page 95), a lift can provide a high level of safety for both your loved one and for your back during transfers. The manual lift is capped rental equipment, so Medicare may cover 80% of the allowed monthly rent for 13 months and then give it to your loved one. Lifts are very durable and sturdy, but you will have to push an air pump handle to raise the lifting arm.

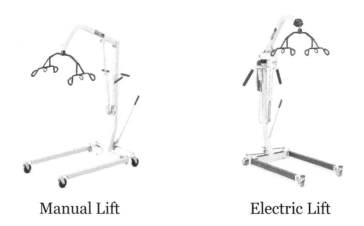

Manual Lift   Electric Lift

What about an electric powered lift?

An electric lift (above right) is similar to a manual lift, except it has an on-board rechargeable battery, which powers an air pump to raise and lower the lifting arm. You can manage well with a manual lift, but if you use a lift multiple times per day, it can require a lot of arm work due to all the pumping.

Can I upgrade from a manual to an electric lift?

Medicare does not cover an electric lift, so first secure Medicare coverage for a capped rental manual lift. Have an electric lift delivered instead and ask the supply company to apply the 13 monthly Medicare rental payments (80% of the allowed amount) for a manual lift toward the purchase price of the electric lift. Your loved one still has to pay 20% of the allowed monthly rental for 13 months and at month 14, will owe the balance of the electric lift purchase price.

What are the limitations of an electric lift?

It doesn't work while plugged in
An electric lift plugs into an outlet for charging, but an electric lift will not operate while plugged in. It doesn't matter if the battery is charged or dead. As long as it is plugged in, it will not operate. This safety feature forces you to unplug the charging cord before you start pushing the wheeled lift around the room.

Usually, there is no manual pump handle
An electric lift usually does not have a manual pump handle to operate the lift arm. If the battery is too weak and needs time to recharge, you can't use the lift until you have enough of a charge in the battery to be able to unplug the charging cord.

If I get an electric lift, should I keep the manual lift as a back up?

If you want the convenience of an electric lift and can afford it, buy one outright, but also take delivery of the Medicare covered manual lift. A manual lift is a reliable back up, because it is very rugged and mechanically simple. An electric lift, although well built, is more complex and may not be available because:

A power failure lasts longer than the battery's remaining charge.

The on-board battery is low or dead, because someone forgot to plug the charging cord in at night or between uses.

The battery or an electrically driven mechanical part fails.

Can I buy a used electric lift?

To save money, buy it used from an original owner who can prove its age and use history. Don't buy used if it has had more than three years of continuous use. Remember, the warranty will probably be expired. On Ebay, search for "patient lift" under Health & Beauty, Medical, Mobility & Disability:

http://health-beauty.shop.ebay.com/items/Medical-Mobility-Disability__WoQQ_catrefZ1QQ_sacatZ11778

On Craigslist: click your city and search for "patient lift".

http://www.craigslist.org/about/sites

How much is a new electric lift and what can I get when I sell it?

Good quality new (on a warranty) electric lifts cost about

$2,000. A couple of years later, it should be easy to sell for about $1,500, which will reduce your net outlay to about $500. Prices vary, so shop the Internet using the keywords: patient lift.

<u>Lift Slings</u>

What is a patient lift sling?

A lift sling is made of durable fabric whose four support straps are looped over four large hooks under the patient lift arm to form a hammock-like fabric chair. After a transfer, the sling stays under your loved one sitting in the wheelchair or on a commode. If you want to use a lift to transfer to a commode, buy a sling with a cutout.

Buy two slings, so you will have a clean and dry one while the other is being washed or is drying. Put them in the washing machine, but not the dryer. Heat and tumbling break down fabric, so put them in the shade to dry. They are super durable, but carefully examine them periodically for wear, especially where the sling loops attach to the main areas of the sling.

There are many types of slings to choose from, so ask your doctor which to buy for your loved one's condition and needs. Medicare doesn't cover slings. Buy the slings new and shop the Internet using the keywords: patient lift sling.

How do I get my loved one into and out of the sling and use the lift?

Get trained first
All methods of transfer require you to be fully trained and educated as to the inherent risks to your loved one and you.

Read the user manual and have a nurse or caregiver train you as the subject and then change places to demonstrate your skills with the trainer in the sling as the subject. The first few times your loved one is transferred with the lift, have an experienced professional helping you. Done properly it is safe, but there are risks of your loved one falling out of the sling and suffering injury or worse if you are not trained or are careless or inattentive while transferring.

Be sure a professional trains and tests you in all specific lift and sling placement methods before you try to use it with your loved one and use only the procedures you learned through professional training.

Wheelchairs

What about wheelchairs?

Standard folding wheelchairs are well made, functional and inexpensive. It is a capped rental item, so Medicare pays 80% of the allowed monthly rent for 13 months and then gives it to your loved one. However, it's not as comfortable as a recliner wheelchair.

When is a basic wheelchair enough?

If your loved one can walk with minimal assistance, a basic wheelchair is needed only after he has stood or walked long enough to become fatigued. If he can sit up with a straight back for long periods without having to be reclined, an upgrade to a recliner wheelchair would be mainly for comfort. In these cases, the basic chair, although not as comfortable, is adequate.

Why should I upgrade to a recliner wheelchair?

Increased comfort and quality of life
If your loved one can't stand in place, walk more than a few steps or walk at all, she will spend a lot of time out of bed in a wheelchair. If there is fatigue after trying to sit up straight, your loved one will feel happier and more comfortable while resting slightly reclined with a straight back.

Sitting up straight
Being out of bed and sitting up straight is important to getting better mentally and physically. We have all felt sorry for someone sitting in a basic chair too fatigued to continue to sit up straight and who is bent forward in an unhealthy posture looking at the ground instead of the world around him.

Wanting to get out and stay out of bed
Being out of bed for as long as possible each day and evening increases the chance for survival and recovery. The more time your loved one spends in bed, the weaker she gets and the harder it is for her to want to get out of bed. Wanting to be out of bed is essential to getting more "vertical", resulting in strengthening and progress.

Keeping the legs comfortably straight
If the legs are not straightened while sitting in the wheelchair, the muscles on the backs of the legs will shorten and become tighter, making it more difficult to try to stand or walk. Passive and active exercise (page 65) and physical therapy is designed to counter weak, tightened and shortened muscles, but straightening the legs while sitting in the wheelchair should be part of the program.

A basic wheelchair with footrests keeps the legs in a bent sitting position. If it has adjustable footrests to straighten the legs, there can still be a strain on your loved one's legs and back if you can't compensate for straighter legs by reclining a little. A recliner wheelchair has detachable and adjustable leg extensions, which can be set from a bent knee position to where the legs are parallel to the floor and straight.

I'm told using a recliner wheelchair will not help my loved one get stronger, because she will not have to try to sit up straight.

Change the angle according to energy level and strength
When your loved one begins sitting in the wheelchair, position the back of the wheelchair to be more vertical. Once she gets fatigued and starts to bend forward, you can recline it according to remaining strength and stamina. Every day there will be varying strength and fatigue, so after making an effort to sit up, she can get a rest break and enjoy life by being more reclined, sitting with a straight back and feeling like part of the group.

A straight-backed wheelchair is an either/or machine
If your loved one has sit up against the vertical back of the wheelchair, then once she is too tired to continue, she'll rest in a bent forward position. Good posture is very important to health and happiness, so after fatigue sets in, it's better to be able to recline enough to achieve a straight back.

Will Medicare cover an upgrade to a recliner wheelchair?

You need to obtain a prescription. It is also a capped rental item, so after 13 months of coverage, your loved one will own it.

What should I ask about recliner wheelchairs?

Ask the home healthcare company to deliver a new wheelchair. You might not get a brand new one, but don't accept a "beater" (worn out). It's best to be the first user, because after 13 months of covered use, your loved one will own it.

Can I buy a recliner wheelchair new?

You can buy one, but regarding this and most Medicare covered capped rental DME, if you buy it outright, Medicare will not cover it.

What safety issues are there with wheelchairs?

Lock the wheels
Always make sure the wheelchair wheels are locked when you do not intend the wheelchair to move. Lock the wheels even on flat surfaces, so you will get into the habit. After locking the wheels, keep an eye on your loved one, because he could unlock the wheels and go for a ride.

Going up and down wheelchair ramps
Always go up and down a ramp with your loved one facing uphill, never downhill, while the back of the wheelchair is vertical. Remember a ramp makes it easier for any wheelchair type to tip backwards. If the wheelchair is a recliner, rent or buy the anti-tip bars (page 106).

Wheelchair Accessories

What are the benefits of various wheelchair accessories?

Common wheelchair accessories include: headrests, removable leg extensions, back cushions, seat cushions, wheelchair trays and for safety, seat belts and anti-tip bars.

Headrest
A detachable headrest extends the back of the wheelchair to support the head when the chair is reclined. It is usually a part of a Medicare covered recliner wheelchair.

Leg extensions
Removable leg extensions are usually part of a Medicare covered recliner wheelchair. They are designed to vary the leg position from bent knees to an elevated position with straight legs (parallel to the floor). Elevating the legs relieves pressure on the lower legs and feet and gives a healthy stretch to the leg muscles on the backs of the legs.

Wheelchair back cushion
The back of the wheelchair is made of a tough fabric, but it usually doesn't come with a back cushion or padding. Your loved one may be more comfortable if you get a foam back cushion with an extra strip of foam for lumbar support (below left). The cushion hangs from two cushion cover straps tied to the upper frame of the wheelchair (below right).

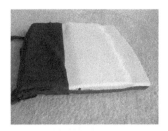
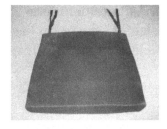

Lumbar Support Strip   Back Cushion w/Cover

How important is the wheelchair seat cushion?

The seat of a wheelchair, which is made of a tough fabric, needs a cushion. Your home healthcare company will include a Medicare provided new foam seat cushion (below left) with the Medicare covered wheelchair. The front view of the cushion (below right) shows the contoured shape of the cushion top.

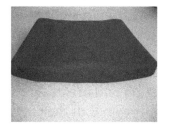 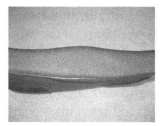

Foam Cushion w/Cover   Front View

The free foam seat cushion is much better than nothing, but it's worthwhile to upgrade it for the following reasons:

To overcome wheelchair seat sag
Wheelchair fabric seats sag from the sides toward the middle, so consider a cushion with a compensating convex bulge on its underside (below). The convex shape ensures the wheelchair seat sag will not cause the top of the cushion to sag as well. It will remain flat like a normal chair seat cushion.

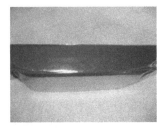

Cushion w/Flat Top And Convex Bottom

To prevent sliding forward in the wheelchair
When sitting in a wheelchair, your loved one can slide
forward on the standard cushion away from the back of
the wheelchair. If the wheelchair back is reclined, he can
slide more easily. As he slides, his back will bend causing
him to slump. Bad posture is hard on the skin, tailbone and
back and can negatively affect digestion and breathing. If
not pulled back up, he could slide all way out of the chair
onto the floor or become compressed against the seat belt.
Repeatedly pulling him back up in the chair will eventually
cause you to strain your back and could lead to your loved
one developing pressure sores due to friction and skin
shearing.

A wedge cushion (below) has a tall front (3 ½" - 5") and a
shorter (1 ½") back. With a wedge shaped cushion, there is
no sliding, because gravity will keep your loved one at the
back of the chair. Because you will not have to repeatedly lift
and pull your loved one in the chair, your loved one's back
and posture will stay straight and your own back will stay
healthy.

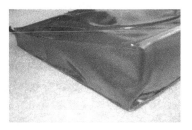

Wedge-Shaped Cushion Tapers
From Front To Back

To increase comfort and better protect the skin
Gel padding (below) is one of many custom cushion top
surfaces designed for comfort and skin protection. Gel
readily adapts to body shape and distributes pressure better
than plain foam. Your loved one will feel more comfortable
and may be able to sit longer without as many skin pressure
problems. No matter how suitable the cushion, you must still
regularly relieve pressure on the sitting area. Ask a nurse
how long your loved one can remain seated in one position
before the risk of pressure sore development increases.

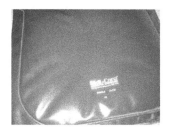

Cushion Top Gel Pocket

How do I choose the right cushion for my loved one?

To select the right cushion, your doctor will consider the
diagnosis, comfort, sensation, skin integrity and history of
skin breakdown, positioning needs, functional and activity

level, type of wheelchair used, client preferences, continence, compliance, cognition, and environment-of-use factors.

Ask your doctor to recommend the cushion type and then compare manufacturers and products to determine which cushion will meet the doctor's recommendation. Search the Internet for manufacturers and vendors using the keywords: wheelchair seat cushions. If in doubt about a final selection, print the information and ask the doctor to review the cushions.

Medicare may cover a cushion upgrade. If so, the cushion type approved will depend on the needs of your loved one as determined by your doctor.

Where can I get more information about a seat cushion with the attributes discussed in this book?

The featured seat cushion is an Ultra Wedge, Gel-Foam Wedge #754180.

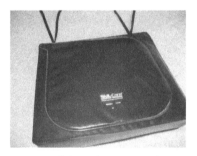
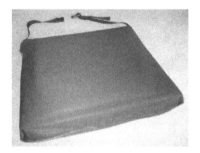

Cushion (no cover)   Cushion w/Cover

For seat cushion product information:

http://www.skil-care.com/cgi-bin/index.cgi?a=fm&p=2012&c=20&prod=754110

For seat cushion vendor ordering and pricing:

http://www.sammonspreston.com/app.aspx?cmd=get_product&id=77532

Wheelchair tray
If you want a tray, you'll have to buy one, so shop the Internet for well made ones at reasonable prices. If you purchase a tray from the home healthcare company supplying the wheelchair, make sure you know in advance what tray you are buying and how much it is. If you are not specific, you might receive a flimsy fiberboard tray and be charged as much as $200! A basic padded vinyl tray (below) with sturdy straps in the $100 price range is adequate for most needs.

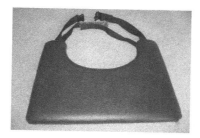

Padded Vinyl Wheelchair Tray

<u>Wheelchair Safety Accessories</u>

Seat belt
Make sure the wheelchair comes with a seat belt. As your loved one gets better, he might suddenly try to get up when you are not looking, which could lead to a fall. The belt doesn't have to be tight to be effective, but when using the belt, keep an eye on your loved one, because if he slides forward on the seat cushion, it can put an unhealthy squeeze on his stomach. A seat belt will stop him from sliding

completely off the chair, but you should also upgrade the seat cushion to a wedge type (pages 102-103) to prevent sliding.

Anti-tip bars
The more reclined the chair position, the less stable it is. Two anti-tip bars (below) slide and snap into the frame at the back of a recliner wheelchair to prevent it from tipping over backwards.

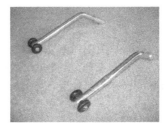

Anti-tip Bars

If, while going up an incline, the chair begins to tip, the wheels at the bottom of the anti-tip bars will touch the ground and restrict the tipping. Instability increases when going up or down a ramp, so keep the back of the chair vertical when using a ramp and always face your loved one uphill.

Medicare covers recliner wheelchairs, but anti-tip bars may not be covered for all chair models, so you may have to purchase the bars.

To view and compare wheelchair accessories by purpose, brand and price:

http://www.sammonspreston.com/app.aspx?cmd=get_
sections&id=100013

Easy To Use Clothing

We are not going to use hospital gowns at home, so what about easy to use clothing?

If pants are difficult to get on and off, order a few pairs of basketball "break away" pants from The NBA Store:

http://www.store.nba.com/home/index.jsp

There are many colors available and they are cool, comfortable and extremely durable. Order them with snaps on the legs and Velcro at the waist and when making the order, specify you do not want pants with zippers, because they slow down clothing changes and can jam or break.

Chapter 5

Extra Equipment At Home

This chapter deals with equipment not covered by Medicare or insurance, but may make your home healthcare experience easier and safer. The equipment includes portable wheelchair ramps, home fire extinguishers and smoke detector/alarms, UPS power systems and household items.

Most of these items are not expensive and some of the longer lasting ones can later be sold used. None can be rented, but you can buy some of them used.

Medical home healthcare companies are set up to bill Medicare and private insurance, so they may not carry all these items. There are great deals from Internet vendors and big box stores.

When considering the purchase of these items, keep in mind Murphy's Law:

"If something can go wrong, it will."

If your loved one uses powered equipment, such as an air pump mattress system and you assume you will not need a back up battery power system (UPS), because you have not had a power outage lately, Murphy's Law can be adapted to:

"If something can go wrong, but has yet to do so, it is probably overdue."

What about portable wheelchair ramps?

A ramp built of wood can warp, snap, bend, become slippery when wet and sag with time. It's not cheap to buy wood and pay a carpenter to build it. For a quick and long lasting solution, buy a portable ramp made of aluminum (below) or fiberglass. They last a long time, are easy to remove and store (they fold up) and you can sell them later. Look on the Internet using the keywords: portable wheelchair ramps.

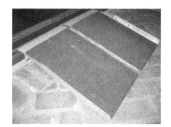 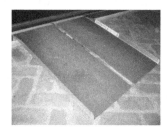

Aluminum Wheelchair Ramps

How do I know what size ramp to buy?

Ramps are made in varying standard lengths of one foot increments and can be purchased over eight feet long. If you buy a long enough ramp, the slope won't be steep, but the longer the ramp, the further out it projects, so keep in mind the maximum amount of room you have. Also, longer ramps can be more easily tripped over.

Discuss the change in elevation (rise) with the vendor customer support person, so you can know the minimum length (run) of ramp you need. This determines the slope of the ramp, which affects safety and the amount of effort you must expend to help your loved one move up the ramp. Be sure to mention the kind of vehicle your loved one is using. It could be a walker, where a standard ramp will suffice, but maybe it should be a bit longer than usual to provide a flatter slope. A wider wheelchair, a heavier person in a sturdier wheelchair or someone using a motorized wheelchair or scooter may need a stronger and wider ramp.

What safety issues are there with ramps?

Visitors and delivery people need to be told the ramp is there and to watch their step, so they don't trip over the fences (guardrails) running the length of each side of the top of the ramp. The fences keep wheelchair wheels from falling off the sides of the ramp and, although they are about 2" high, they are not easy to see. As you point out the ramp, kick the side of a fence to draw attention to it.

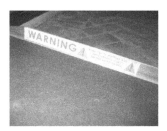

Ramp Section Showing Side Fence
(notice the trip-warning label)

Always take a wheelchair up and down a ramp with your loved one facing uphill. Make sure the back of a recliner wheelchair is vertical, so the wheelchair is as stable as it can be. The recliner wheelchair must have anti-tip bars attached. Make sure the seat belt is secure and your loved one's feet are on the footrests and not dragging on the ground. Before you start down a ramp, look behind you and watch your step, so you and your loved one don't fall with the wheelchair and your loved one falling on you.

<u>Fire Safety</u>

If I smell smoke or see a fire, I'll just call 911, right?

You are responsible for your loved one, who may be immobile or have limited mobility, so always call 911 without delay. But you should have smoke detector/alarms, so if a fire occurs, you will discover it as soon as possible and get your loved one to safety sooner.

Do your best to prevent fires. If there is medical equipment at home, like oxygen equipment with its own specific fire hazards and fire safety precautions, go over them with the technician delivering and setting up the oxygen equipment (Chapter 7).

What about fire safety equipment?

Get a couple of small fire extinguishers and smoke particle/ carbon monoxide (CO) detector/alarms. CO from fire or exhaust is colorless, odorless and deadly.

What should I know about fire extinguishers and the smoke detector?

Keep fire extinguishers available
Get at least two and keep them in your loved one's room. If one doesn't work or if it runs out, you'll have another. Make sure everyone knows where the extinguishers are and how to use them. Don't let anyone move them from the room or put them in the room where they can't be seen.

Smoke and CO can persist
When the smoke detector (below) senses smoke particles or carbon monoxide (CO), it sounds an alarm.

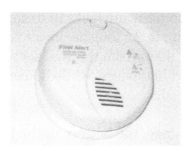

Smoke And CO Detector/Alarm

You may not have a fire, but the CO alarm may sound. If someone nearby uses a gasoline-powered machine, like a chain saw, you'll close the windows to keep out the noise, but harmful CO from exhaust can accumulate and remain under roof eaves. When you reopen the windows, the CO can drift into the room. Close the windows and open another door or window on another side of the residence. If the alarm doesn't stop, you may need to move your loved one.

If the smoke detector/alarm is battery powered (not powered by house wiring), it usually uses a 9-volt battery.

Electric Power Outages

What can I do about electric power outages?

If you have power outages or brief "brownouts", you may need back up power, such as an Uninterrupted Power Supply (UPS) for your home healthcare medical devices.

What is a UPS?

A UPS is a power monitoring and self-charging battery system. It reacts instantly when the power to the home stops and its battery automatically kicks in to supply power to the devices plugged into it. As long as power is supplied to the home, the current flows from the wall socket through the UPS to the plugged in devices, while it keeps its on-board battery fully charged.

During a power outage, the battery in the UPS supplies power to the devices plugged into its sockets. When the power returns, the UPS switches back to standby mode, letting the current flow through it to the plugged in devices and begins charging its battery for the next outage.

What should I know about a UPS?

A UPS is automatic and doesn't need maintenance. The length of time the battery will supply power during a power outage depends on the UPS battery capacity and the number and type of devices you plug into the UPS. The more electric current the UPS battery has to deliver, the faster the battery will drain. Although the rechargeable battery lasts a long time, it has to be replaced eventually, so if you later sell the UPS used, you won't get much.

A UPS is easy to set up. If you buy from a large, well-known company, you can call the phone number listed on its website and ask their technical support group about the set up.

Which devices should be plugged into the UPS?

If you have a continuous low air loss mattress (LAL) (page 87) or an alternating air pressure pad (APP) (page 89), plug in the air pump, because the LAL air pump and the APP air pump do not have back up batteries and during an outage, the mattress or pad will go flat.

Tube feeding pumps (page 190) and portable suction machines (page 150) have on-board rechargeable batteries, so if power is lost, they can last an hour or more on their own. If you plug them into the UPS, they will not start to draw from their own batteries until after the UPS battery is depleted, but the UPS will run out of power sooner.

How can I get a UPS?

Buy one before you bring your loved one home. American Power Conversion (APC) is a well-regarded brand.

http://www.apcc.com/products/category.cfm?id=13&subid=5

<u>Household Appliances And Tools</u>

Any other appliances or tools you recommend?

Fax machine
This is useful for receiving written or printed documents from healthcare professionals. You may need to send documents or copies you have received to others involved with the case or to billing departments and insurance companies. A fax machine will greatly help you manage your loved one's case.

If you have a landline, you don't need an extra landline, because many fax machines can recognize a fax instead of a voice call coming in. If you have only a cell phone, you will have to get a landline for the fax.

Mini microwave
A small unit costs about $60 and will enable you to quickly and easily heat water and food near your loved one.

Cube refrigerator
A mini fridge costs under $100 and can be used to hold "Keep Refrigerated" medicines near the bedside and food near the microwave.

A short sturdy stepladder
If you have an old, unstable stepladder, get a new one and insist everyone use the new stepladder to reach for things. To prevent falls, have each person demonstrate its use. No standing on chairs or furniture.

Flashlights And Batteries

What about flashlights and batteries?

Flashlights
Keep a flashlight by your bed and another one by the bed of your loved one. D or C size batteries are for the larger flashlights and AA or AAA sizes are for penlights. Keep a lot of spares. Buy your batteries in bulk to save money and store them in the refrigerator for a long shelf life.

Don't use candles. They can dry out the room air, cause a fire, blow out and don't give directional light. If you have supplemental oxygen (Chapter 7) in the home, never use matches or candles, because of the likelihood of an explosion.

Chapter 6

Staying Organized At Home

Your advocacy helped make the most of your loved one's hospital stay and the benefits of your effort will continue with home healthcare. Your loved is safely home, but the attention of the hospital has been replaced by a near absence of health care support at home.

Quiet, isn't it?

This chapter will help you organize common daily healthcare tasks at home, coordinate the care of your loved one and manage the appointments of visiting medical providers, such as visiting nurses, physical therapists and mobile X-ray companies.

The doctor will usually order laboratory tests to diagnose, treat and assess your loved one. There are actions you can take to expedite and confirm laboratory analysis results for blood and other samples taken by visiting nurses get to the doctor who ordered them. The more relevant and accurate information you can provide doctors and nurses, the better the care your loved one will receive.

<u>Keeping Tasks Organized</u>

How do I begin to coordinate everyone helping out?

Make a cheat sheet of the daily routine and give copies to family members and others helping out. Outline your loved one's daily schedule and list her likes and dislikes. Include preferred methods to perform tasks like answering the door and the phone, taking messages, accepting deliveries and other everyday occurrences. Include your cell number, so anyone filling in can find you quickly.

What is an easy way to make sure everyone helping out stays informed?

Get a white board with erasable marking pens. Hang it on the wall near the bed, so everyone can see it. It's great to announce messages and alerts, such as:

Antibiotic started/ending	(days/dates)
Visiting nurse coming	(time/day/date)
Medicine delivery due by	(time/day/date)
Supplies ordered and quantity	(order date, delivery date)

With so much to do each day, how can I organize my tasks?

The more you do each day and the longer you have to care for your loved one, the more valuable is a properly created list to manage the case. You need more than just a daily To Do list. You want to create a reference journal to easily recall events or information days, weeks or months later.

What's the best way to keep a journal?

Use a computer and a word processing program. From the first day forward, append each date to the last and keep scrolling further down the same document. This way, you can either scroll back into the recent past to see what still needs to be done or, if you need to locate something further back and you can't remember the date of the event, you can do a keyword search to find it quickly.

How can I make my journal easy to use?

Use color
When you are making entries into the journal, highlight in red things remaining to be done. When you scroll back to past days, it is easy to see items still left to do. After taking care of them, change the red text highlights to black.

Pull excerpts to make a daily To Do list
Copy and paste all the red items from past days onto a daily To Do list. Print and use it as a check off list during the day. As you take care of these tasks, check them off with a pen and as new items come up, write them in with a pen.

At the end of the day, update the journal
The daily To Do list can be used to update the computerized journal. If there are new, but not yet completed items jotted down during the day on the list, add them to the journal and highlight them in red. In the journal, change from red to black any items completed. In the morning, you can print out a new list.

Managing Visiting Medical Providers

Usually, a visiting nurse, physical therapist or X-ray

technician will show up at a residence on time, perform medical or technical services without difficulty and where necessary, follow up with the laboratory or doctor. However, there are commonly occurring problems related to home visits and if you are aware of them ahead of time, you can help head them off. The rest of this chapter will alert you to these minor difficulties and will specify actions you can take before, during and after visits to help make sure the visits, medical tasks performed and follow ups stay on track.

Visiting Nurse Appointment Tips

How can I "back-stop" regularly scheduled nurse visits?

Call the day before the visit
If you call the agency the day before the scheduled visit, you can double-check to see if a nurse who visits regularly is scheduled the next day. If a usual nurse is not available due to illness or vacation, a substitute nurse might not be aware she is scheduled to handle your visit. Get her cell number from the agency, put it in your journal and call her to verify she knows to come and ask her when she will be there. If the agency won't provide her cell number, ask them to call the nurse and request she call you to confirm.

Call the morning of the visit
If the nurse is running late and has not called to let you know she is coming, call the agency, so they can have as much notice as possible to find her or schedule someone else to visit. Nurses get sick, take vacations, quit or swap days, but new schedule information isn't always shared. Get all your visiting nurses' cell numbers and put them in your journal (page 119), so you can call them directly if there seems to be a problem.

What additional issues are there with nurse visits?

Your loved one is a "hard stick"
If there is no intravenous (IV) line, the nurse has to "stick" by inserting a needle, usually into the arm. If your loved one is a "hard stick", it means she has difficult-to-find blood vessels.

A visiting nurse is restricted to a maximum number of stick attempts (typically three) per visit. Ask the agency, which of their nurses have the most success with "hard stick" cases and ask them to be scheduled. Also request the nurses bring butterfly needles (below), which are thinner needles used for children and adults with hard to find veins, have plastic connections for easy gripping and stay in the vein better than regular needles. If a nurse is having a hard time, suggest she use a warm compress to bring the veins up.

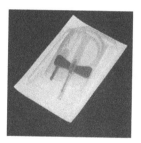

Butterfly Needle

Request early morning nurse visits (page 62), so it's still early enough to get another nurse to your home to attempt to get the blood.

If, after an unsuccessful visit, the agency says there is no one else available, request a phlebotomist. This is a technician who only does blood draws and can get blood from anyone.

FYI, the term "hard stick" is slang to describe a person difficult to draw blood from. Some nurses don't like the term, but it does get the meaning across in fewer words.

The nurse cancels or doesn't show up and the agency says they have no available nurses
If it's a regularly scheduled visit, call the doctor and ask if he needs the laboratory analysis done today or if it can wait until tomorrow. If he needs it today, ask him to fax a STAT (urgent) order to the nurse agency. Call them to be sure they received it. The agency will find a nurse.

There is an urgent request for an additional visit
If there is a change in the medical condition of your loved one, the doctor may order a STAT (urgent) visit, but what if the agency can't get a nurse to the residence soon enough? Call another Medicare certified agency and ask if they have a nurse who can come on short notice. If your loved one is a "hard stick" patient (page 121), be sure to mention it.

The doctor's office must fax an order to the alternate agency for the visit. If the nurse is not from your usual agency or from your hospital home healthcare department, once she obtains needed samples, you may have to take them to the hospital laboratory.

The laboratory is closed
You might have to drop off a blood, urine or sputum sample, so ask ahead of time where the laboratory drop-off desk is and the hours it is open (Appendix 1). Ask where to park nearby and if there is a free 10-20 minute parking zone. If the usual drop-off location is closed, ask for the location of the laboratory inside the hospital. At least one hospital laboratory location is open 24 hours a day, 365 days a year.

Nurse visits need periodic certification to continue
At least every 60 days, Medicare requires your loved one to be re-certified by the Home Health Agency (HHA) for nurse visits to continue for the next 60 days. A visiting nurse does this routine paperwork.

Ask the nurse about re-certification
Ask the nurse her opinion about continued visits and when the next re-certification is needed. If a visiting nurse discharges (doesn't re-certify and ends the nurse visits) your loved one without telling you, when you call the agency the day before the next visit to confirm it, you will be told the visits are over. You will have to call the doctor and get a new standing order faxed to the agency and the next visiting nurse will have to complete the paperwork to re-start the visits for another 60 days.

<u>Arranging Additional Nurse Visits</u>

We need an additional (unscheduled) nurse visit.

When there is the urgent need for a blood, sputum or urine sample for laboratory analysis or because of pain issues, high temperature or a change in behavior, the doctor may make an additional nurse visit request. For a visit on short notice, ask the nursing agency if the doctor must also write STAT (urgent) on the faxed order.

What can I do to keep an additional visit on track?

Call the agency to verify:

- They received the faxed visitation order
- The order has the required information
- The visit is actually scheduled

- The scheduled time of the visit
- The name of the nurse scheduled to visit

The visiting nurse during the additional visit says she will relay my loved one's information to the nurse who usually visits.

Follow up by calling the intended recipient to confirm the communication was made. Remember to use your journal to record this and all events. When the usual nurse visits the next time, refer to your journal to recall the information.

Visiting Physical Therapy Tips

The visiting therapist says, "Your loved one is not responding fast enough to therapy", so he can't re-certify her for Medicare covered future visits.

Generally, rehabilitation potential is considered "progress" and progress is a criterion for continuing (re-certification for another 60 days) Medicare covered physical therapy (and other types of therapy) visits.

If the visiting therapist is passive, uninspired or not motivating or is going through the motions in a very emotionally detached, impersonal way, your loved one might not respond as expected. If you don't think the therapist is working out, call the agency to send someone else.

We are being told, "She doesn't want to do her physical therapy".

It's easy to blame the patient without trying to find a reason for a lack of participation. If your loved one demonstrates an unwillingness or inability to participate in therapy, watch for physical discomfort, pain, fatigue or an emotional reason.

What are some common reasons for not participating in physical therapy?

Ask your loved one how she feels. Your loved one could be tired, depressed, afraid, not feeling well, in pain or begin to feel pain during therapy. Antibiotics or other medicines could be dragging her down.

You know your loved one better than a therapist, so make the therapist aware of your loved one's likes and dislikes. Some people like to be touched while exercising and some don't, so it could be the interaction or lack thereof. Maybe she doesn't like or relate to the physical therapist and another person can motivate her.

A weak and disoriented person can still be quite perceptive, so if the physical therapist does not seem committed or doesn't relate to your loved one, your loved one may not commit or fully participate.

Can music help with healing and recovery and motivate my loved one to exercise?

Music can relax, motivate and make people happier and more hopeful. A study, cited in Appendix 4, concluded music helps brain function improve after a stroke, especially if the music is included with other therapies and starts soon after the stroke.

Try music from your loved one's youth to make the therapy more fun and motivating. Your loved one may react to a favorite song by exercising longer and more vigorously. She might forget how hard she is working while she is exercising.

If the rehabilitation department doesn't offer music, bring your own music device and a couple of speakers. If your loved one does therapy at home, play music during exercise sessions.

Bose and other audio companies make compact, high quality stand-alone speakers for about $80 a pair, so even at low volume, they sound great. You can get them at a big box store or online.

Mobile X-ray Visit Tips

How can I help keep the X-ray appointment and results on track?

Make sure they have received the faxed prescription
The doctor's office needs to fax to the company a prescription specifying the X-rays. If you have a fax machine, ask the doctor's office to fax you a copy as well. If the X-ray company office tells you they didn't get the fax, you can send it without having to bother the doctor.

Request an estimated time of arrival (ETA)
When you call the company to confirm they received the fax, get an ETA for the visit and ask the name and cell phone number of the technician dispatched.

Always request an ETA when scheduling and then waiting for time sensitive events, such as other tests, deliveries and nurse visits. This will keep you involved if an event falls behind schedule and can help you schedule events, so they best fit your loved one's daily routine.

Call to update the ETA
About an hour before the ETA, call the technician on his cell

to see if he is running on time. Ask him where he his and if you are the next appointment.

Make sure the radiologist's report is faxed to the doctor
After the X-rays are taken, the technician will fill out forms for you to sign. Get copies and make sure the technician writes the ordering doctor's fax number on the forms, so the ordering doctor can later receive a faxed copy of the X-ray results from the radiologist. Call the doctor's office later in the day, but well before closing time to find out if the faxed results have been received (and what they were). Ask the doctor's office how late you can call them to confirm receipt. If they stop answering the phone at 6 P.M., call them by 5:30 P.M.

Get the radiologist's contact information
Before the X-ray technician leaves the residence, ask the technician for the radiologist's business hours and after-hours phone numbers, because if by the end of the day the doctor has not heard from the radiologist or received a fax, the doctor will need to call the radiologist for the opinion.

When you call the doctor's office to find out if they have received the opinion, but are told they are still waiting, give them the radiologist's phone numbers and then call the radiologist to let him know the doctor will be calling.

You may have to make more follow up calls
If the doctor does not receive the results before his office closes, call the radiologist and let him know you are trying to find the doctor, so they can discuss the X-rays. If you have a fax machine, ask the radiologist to fax the opinion to you. If it is after hours, find the doctor or a colleague on duty at the hospital and tell him the opinion is ready. The doctor may ask you to read the opinion over the phone.

Laboratory Test Tips

When the doctor orders a blood sample, a visiting nurse may take it with her for delivery to the laboratory. There are various reasons a laboratory will reject a blood sample. They are listed below, so you can take action to help avoid a sample rejection.

Why does the laboratory reject the samples?

The sample volume is insufficient
If the blood volume in a tube is too small, the laboratory will reject the sample. Ask the visiting nurse if she is getting enough blood per tube. If not, ask her to draw another sample, but if your loved one is difficult to draw from, request another nurse to come and try.

The sample is too old
If blood samples are not delivered to the laboratory soon enough after being drawn, the laboratory will reject them. Ask the visiting nurse how long is allowed from the time of the blood draw to the laboratory.

If you are delivering samples to the laboratory, but you can't leave right away, put the tubes containing the samples in the fridge, not the freezer. When you leave, put some dry paper towels around the tubes and put the wrapped tubes in a cup of ice cubes and wrap the cup and ice with foil for the ride. Put this in a large zip lock bag with a copy of the doctor's laboratory order.

The wrong tube (cap color) was used
The blood flows into specialized vacuum tubes, which resemble small test tubes with colored caps (below). Each vacuum tube and cap color is specific to a type of analysis.

If a wrong color tube is used, the laboratory will reject the sample. If the visiting nurse is from your hospital home healthcare department, she will probably know the hospital laboratory's tube color requirements. If she is from an outside agency, she might not know, so ask her. If she is not sure, call the hospital laboratory or the hospital home healthcare department and find out.

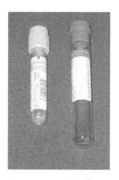

Vacuum Tubes

Visiting nurses are supposed to make sure there is a complete supply of all required tubes at the residence, but learn what the tubes look like and keep track of the supply on hand, so you don't run out. Write it in your journal for future reference.

The tube is expired
Vacuum tubes have expiration dates and if the laboratory receives an expired tube, they will reject the sample. Even if there is a complete supply of all required tubes at the residence, make a note of their expiration dates, so you can request from visiting nurses more tubes well before they expire.

Is there a way to make sure the right colored tubes are available?

Ask a visiting nurse to bring at least one spare set of tubes (below) with cap colors specified by the laboratory. Look at the tube expiration dates to be sure they are still good and are not about to expire.

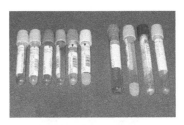

Vacuum Tube Assortment

What can I do to make sure the doctor gets the laboratory report?

Call the doctor's office later in the afternoon and ask if they received the laboratory report. If not, ask the doctor's office how late you can call them to confirm receipt. If they stop answering the phone at 6 P.M., call them by 5:30 P.M.

Keep in mind, someone (usually the visiting nurse) has to take the sample to the laboratory and the laboratory needs a few hours to analyze it and generate a report. If the analysis involves growing a culture, the laboratory report could take a few days.

Making Time To Exercise And Relax

What are some of the best ways to relax?

Take daily walks
Get out and walk in a relaxing setting. It is more beneficial if you walk with a supportive friend with a positive attitude.

Swim
Swimming and treading water for 15 minutes a day is great exercise and is very relaxing. If you don't have a pool, join a gym with a pool or go to the local YMCA. Swimming will put you around people having fun, which can help take your mind off your stressful situation.

Meditate
Find a quiet place to lie down and breathe slowly and deeply for 20 minutes. You can fall asleep, so set an alarm if you need to wake up by a certain time.

Once a month, get a massage
A large part of caregiver stress is doing for others without a break and feeling unappreciated. A massage will alleviate harmful stress and help prevent muscle strain and other stress related illnesses. Think of a massage and the previously mentioned suggestions as medicinal, not as luxuries, because stress absorbed and not released can accumulate and cause illness.

Chapter 7

Oxygen Equipment And Respiratory Issues

Supplemental oxygen is commonly needed during hospital stays, recovery at home and longer-term for chronic medical and respiratory problems.

If your loved one needs oxygen equipment at home, ask the nurses at the hospital for training in the use of the equipment, measuring blood oxygen levels and oxygen use precautions.

This chapter gives tips to help you understand the nature and use of home healthcare oxygen equipment such as oxygen bottles and oxygen concentrators.

Keeping the room temperature and humidity in the optimal range and keeping the room air clean may be beneficial to your loved one's ability to continue to breathe properly.

Additional home healthcare devices that aid breathing are also discussed, such as mist machines, consumer humidifiers and air purifiers.

<u>Oxygen Equipment And Supplies</u>

What are the basics of oxygen bottles?

Full oxygen bottles (below left) are delivered and exchanged for empties with at least one removable regulator (below center). The regulator adjusts to control the rate of oxygen delivered per minute in 1, 2, 3... liter increments. It has an analog (needle) gauge (below right) to show the amount of oxygen left in the bottle.

Post the doctor's order for the supplemental (more than room air) oxygen rate, so the regulator is always set at the ordered number. Every time oxygen is used, check the regulator setting number to make sure the rate is correct and check the gauge to be sure there is plenty of oxygen left in the bottle. Check the regulator gauge level periodically and change the bottle for a full one as soon as the gauge indicates a low oxygen level.

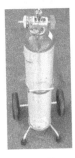 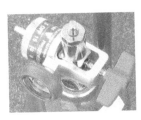 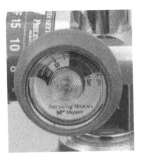

Oxygen Bottle   Oxygen Regulator   Regulator Gauge

Be familiar with the operation of the regulator and how to use the oxygen bottle valve wrench (below) to open and close the bottle pressure valve, which sends pressure to the regulator. The healthcare company supplying the oxygen should give you at least one when they deliver and set up the home oxygen equipment. Hang the wrench on a hook above the oxygen bottle by the bed. Request a spare wrench, store it in a safe place and put a note on the wall saying where the spare is kept.

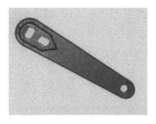

Oxygen Bottle Valve Wrench

Oxygen Bottle Tips

How do I change an oxygen bottle?

As you should with all new equipment and procedures, have a professional (in this case, the technician setting up the home oxygen) train and allow you time to demonstrate you can effectively perform each newly learned task from memory. Take as much time as you need to repeat each task a minimum of three times or until you feel like it is automatic. Take notes for your journal.

Use the bottle valve wrench to close the bottle valve supplying pressure to the regulator, remove the regulator, put the regulator on a full bottle and use the wrench to open the bottle pressure valve to the regulator. When not in use, make sure the regulator is off (set at zero), so you won't drain the new bottle after the wrench opens the pressure valve to the regulator. Remember to look at the regulator gauge to verify the new bottle is full, not just partially filled or empty.

Can I use the bottle wrench to open the bottle valve instead of turning the regulator dial to start the oxygen flowing?

Don't use the wrench to open or close the bottle pressure valve to the regulator, unless you are changing to a new bottle. Keep in mind, when the bottle pressure valve is closed, the regulator gauge will show EMPTY, even on a full bottle!

Leave the bottle pressure valve open to the regulator and turn the regulator dial to zero when the bottle in not in use. When you turn the regulator dial to start the oxygen, the oxygen will start flowing quickly at the proper setting and the gauge will always show the true amount of oxygen left in the bottle.

Common Mistakes With Oxygen Bottles

What are some common mistakes made with oxygen bottles?

The actual oxygen level of the bottle will not show on the regulator gauge unless the bottle pressure valve is opened to the regulator.

Starting a new bottle low on oxygen
Don't assume the new bottle is full. After you attach the regulator to the new bottle, use the wrench to open the bottle pressure valve to the regulator and check the oxygen level gauge. If the level is low on the new bottle, mark it as empty and try another one.

The gauge shows EMPTY, but the bottle is full
Don't assume the current bottle is empty. If a bottle you

haven't used for awhile has a valve gauge showing EMPTY, use the bottle wrench to check to be sure the bottle pressure valve to the regulator is open.

Not being aware of or following safety precautions
Oxygen equipment should never be used around an open flame or anything producing sparks, because pure oxygen is extremely flammable and there could be an explosion and fire. The tall cylindrical bottles should always be secured, so they can't tip over or roll around. Ask the technician delivering the equipment to go over safety precautions with you, take notes for your journal and post them where everyone can see them.

Oxygen Concentrator Basics

What is an oxygen concentrator?

Room air at sea level is about 21% oxygen and 78% nitrogen. The oxygen (O2) concentrator (below left) takes in room air and concentrates it to higher oxygen level by removing from it a set amount of nitrogen. The concentrated oxygen/air mixture is sent through a tube to a patient.

There is a shelf on the concentrator to attach an optional plastic water humidifier bottle (below right), so you can adjust the moisture content of the delivered air. The concentrator has a regulator dial with the same numbered oxygen flow rate settings as an oxygen bottle regulator. As with the bottles, pay attention to the ordered oxygen level setting to be sure it is always set as ordered.

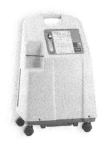 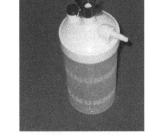

O2 Concentrator   Humidifier

Do I need a concentrator if I have plenty of oxygen bottles? Will Medicare cover it if I have bottles?

Bottles are handy for portability and power outages, so use the concentrator when possible to conserve the bottles. During a power outage or if the concentrator stops working, you will need to switch to a full oxygen bottle with an attached tube to a face mask, tracheal mask or nose canula. Medicare may cover a concentrator even if you have bottles.

Oxygen Concentrator Tips

What else should I ask about the concentrator?

When running, a concentrator makes a low level bass sound, so put it in a far corner of the room and ask for a long enough oxygen tube to reach your loved one.

Ask how often the technician will visit the residence to check the machine. The technician also services the internal air filter. Ask about the service schedule for the internal and external air filters and if you are responsible for any maintenance, like cleaning the external filter.

How can I know if the concentrator is working properly?

Ask the technician delivering and setting up the oxygen equipment what visual and audible alarms are built into the concentrator to alert you if it is not producing an adequate level of concentrated oxygen. Learn the normal sound of the machine (usually a low level bass) when it is running properly, so you can recognize a potential problem if it sounds different.

How do I know the oxygen connections are tight?

When using an oxygen bottle or concentrator, check the connections by feeling for air pressure coming out of the patient end of the delivery tube. If there is little or no pressure, either the oxygen source is shut off, not working or there is a leak along the air tube pathway.

Medicare covers durable medical equipment rental for 13 months, except oxygen equipment?

Your loved one will own Medicare capped rental DME (page 79) after 13 continuous months of covered rental, but will own capped rental oxygen equipment after 36 continuous months of covered rental.

Humidity Issues

Why is optimal humidity important?

Too low
Low room humidity dries the lungs, making it difficult to form and cough up mucus. People recovering from illness need to keep their lungs clear, but as accumulating mucus

in the lungs becomes drier, it gets thicker and stickier. This makes it harder to expel mucus and breathe properly and can provide an opportunity for infection. Low humidity also makes people throw off body heat faster, which makes them feeling chilled at temperatures they normally prefer.

Too high
Regardless of room temperature, if the humidity is high, people can't throw off body heat as fast as they can in lower humidity. Recovering and elderly people have a harder time reacting to temperature changes, so higher humidity levels can make them uncomfortable and cause their body temperatures to increase.

How can using a heater or air conditioner affect humidity?

Winters in many places have low humidity and running the heater or using a fireplace will further dry out room air.

In summer, high temperatures and/or high humidity make it difficult for a recovering or elderly person trying to stay cool, especially if running a fever. Running an air conditioner (A/C) can bring the temperature and humidity down to a more comfortable level, but A/C can excessively dry out room air.

There is an ideal zone of humidity and temperature, so as you use a heater or air conditioner to keep the temperature range on target for your loved one, remember the humidity may drop below what is best for your loved one's medical condition.

Mist Machine Basics

Is there a machine designed to humidify room air and deliver it via an air hose to my loved one?

A specialized mist machine compressor (below left) forces room air through a pipe (below center) into an attached hanging water bottle humidifier (below right), so it will bubble through and exit as humidified air. You can set the moisture level by turning a plastic dial on the water bottleneck. A humidifier hose is attached to the water bottle to send the moisturized air to your loved one. It provides a much more sudden, intense and extended dose of humidified air to a dry throat and lungs than a consumer humidifier can.

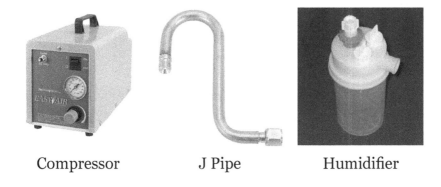

Compressor   J Pipe   Humidifier

For more information about this equipment:

http://www.precisionmedical.com/index.asp?Product=Compressors&Item=EasyAir

What should I request with the mist machine?

Request a humidifier hose adapter (below left) to be able to attach an oxygen (O2) tube to send oxygen from an oxygen bottle or concentrator while the mist machine is running.

Ask the oxygen technician to train you and make sure you take the time to demonstrate to the technician you can set it up and make it work.

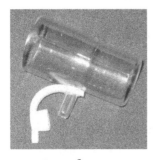
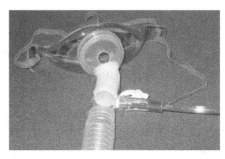

O2 Adapter   Mask, Hose, O2 Adapter, O2 Tube

One end of the adapter goes into the humidifier hose and the other end of the adapter attaches to the face or tracheal mask. The adapter's small side port (above left) accepts the slimmer oxygen delivery tube (above right).

Make sure you receive a couple of mist condensation bags (below), so condensation in the humidifier hose can be collected and easily drained. Otherwise, accumulating water in the hose will start to interfere with humidified air flowing from the humidifier bottle to your loved one.

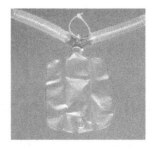

Condensation Collection/Drain Bag

What about changing the hoses and maintaining the mist machine?

The technician setting up the equipment should give you a box of coiled hose you can measure and cut with a pair of scissors when you need to replace the humidifier hose sections. This is considered disposable equipment, because it gets contaminated with use and must be replaced on a regular schedule. Ask the technician about recommended schedules for replacing disposables like the hose sections and the mist condensation bag. Ask where the compressor air filters are located and if you or the technician cleans/replaces them, how to clean or replace them and how often.

What about Medicare coverage for oxygen equipment and mist machine disposable supplies?

Medicare covers disposable supplies for covered oxygen equipment and a mist machine. This includes tubes to deliver oxygen from an oxygen bottle or an oxygen concentrator to other covered disposables such as face masks (covering the nose and mouth), tracheal masks (covering the tracheostomy, a surgically created hole in the throat to allow air to pass) and nose canulas (tubes branching to each nostril). Also included are the humidifier bottles, humidifier hoses and mist condensation bags.

Room Humidifiers

What about consumer humidifiers?

A consumer humidifier (below left) is handy to maintain the humidity of an average sized room, so you won't have to use the noisier mist machine compressor and its cumbersome humidifier hose as often. However, if your loved one has a medical condition causing his lungs and throat to become too dry even when the room humidity is adequate, you may need to run the compressor for brief periods as a regular mist therapy. Medicare doesn't cover consumer humidifiers.

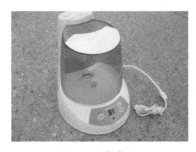
Humidifier

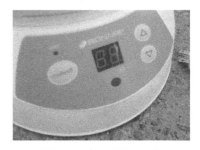
Humistat Display

Can a consumer humidifier sense the room humidity and be set to start when the humidity is too low and stop when the humidity becomes adequate?

Not all have a humistat, so ask before you buy. If so, the humidifier control panel/display (above right) makes it easy to set the humidity to the preferred range of 35%-50%. A humistat sensor switches the heating element on when the humidity drops below the low setting (35%) and shuts it off above the high setting (50%).

Why is 35%-50% the desired humidity range?

Humidity under 30% is too dry. A recovering person needs adequate moisture to help prevent the thickening of mucus in the lungs, so it can be formed and coughed up. Low humidity also makes people feel cooler than the actual room temperature and dries the skin and eyes. Above 50% for long periods is too wet. A humid room can create condensation on the windows and other cool surfaces and harbor mold, mildew, dust mites and bacteria. High humidity makes people feel warmer than the actual room temperature and makes it harder for everyone to throw off body heat and stay cool. Temporary spikes and dips above and below the preferred range are not a problem.

What is the downside to room humidifiers?

You can't just set it and forget it. As it sends moisture into the air, the water level in the tank drops. It will shut off if the water level gets too low, so you have to monitor the water level or the machine will not continue to turn on when more humidity is needed. You also need to clean the humidifier after each use to prevent mold or bacterial growth inside the machine and around the heating element. Bacteria or mold growth in the humidifier can be dispersed into the room air with the moisture emitted. Be sure to read the user manual to learn about recommended cleaning procedures.

What else I should buy with a humidifier?

It's a good idea to buy a temperature/humidity display with large numbers (below), because when you know the humidity of the room, you can set up the humidifier only when necessary. You can get one at a local drugstore.

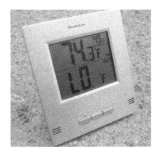

Temp/Humidity Display (showing 74 F. and 49%)

<u>Air Purifiers</u>

Should I consider air purifiers?

People with asthma, allergies, tracheostomies, respiratory diseases and respiratory conditions are sensitive to air quality. There is a debate between researchers, allergists, consumer groups and manufacturers of air purifiers about which type works best. Here is a website to research purifier types, room volume capacities, features, test results, prices and to read reviews:

http://www.air-purifiers-america.com/

What kinds of air purifiers are there?

Ionic
Ionic air purifiers use electrostatic (charged) metal plates to attract and hold onto air borne particles. They don't use a fan, so they are silent and don't use much electricity. They are easy to maintain, because you just wipe off the metal surfaces. They don't use disposable filters, so they cost much less to operate.

High Efficiency Particulate Air (HEPA)
HEPA purifiers (below left) use a fan to draw air through their filters, so you can hear them running and they consume more power than the ionic. HEPA has two filters: a disposable charcoal filter (center) wrapped around the outside of the round HEPA filter (below right). The charcoal filter should be very dirty at each monthly changing, which is evidence the unit is cleaning the air. After about three years, the HEPA filter should be replaced. In my opinion, as long as you regularly change the charcoal filter, HEPA is much more effective.

146

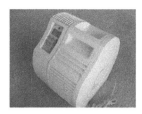 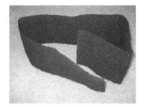 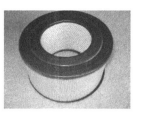

HEPA Purifier   Charcoal Filter   HEPA Filter
                            Strip

Where do I get replacement charcoal filters?

The charcoal air filter has a part number related to the model number of the air purifier. For good deals on air filters:

http://www.filtersnow.com

Chapter 8

Suction Machines And Equipment Troubleshooting

If your loved one has trouble swallowing or has a tracheostomy (a surgically created hole in the throat to allow air to pass), chances are respiratory (airway and lung) suctioning will be part of ongoing home healthcare. Suctioning is usually done at the hospital by a respiratory therapist or nurse, but at home, you may have to perform suctioning and train others to fill in for you.

Ask nurses at the hospital for training. Practice suctioning techniques in front of the nurses, so you can demonstrate your ability and show an understanding of related lung and respiratory issues. Nurses can also give you training in measuring blood oxygen and giving supplemental oxygen.

Ask the home healthcare supply company technician delivering and setting up the bedside suction equipment to show you how to use, clean and troubleshoot it.

The two most typical home healthcare suction machines are described, so the troubleshooting tips offered should apply to most home bedside suction equipment.

<u>Suction Machines</u>

What are home suction machines?

A home suction machine, called an aspirator, creates a
mild reverse pressure (suction), so a connected catheter (a
disposable, sterile, narrow, flexible tube) can pull mucus
out of the lungs, throat or the mouth when a person can't
cough it all the way up or spit it out. Your loved one may be
too weak to bring up thickening or massive mucus from her
lungs. Suctioning the lungs helps breathing and clears the
mouth and throat of mucus to prevent accumulation and
choking. The suctioned liquid goes into a plastic catch jar,
which is emptied and cleaned a few times each day.

What kinds of home suction machines are there?

Medicare covers two suction machines
One stationary and one portable suction machine are covered
as capped rental (page 79), so after 13 months of continuous
rental, your loved one will own them.

Stationary vs. portable
The stationary machine (below left) is used at the bedside
and must be plugged in. There is no battery, so it will not
operate during a power outage. The portable (below right)
plugs in for power and to charge its on-board battery, which
comes in handy during power outages and trips away from
available electric power. Keep the portable plugged in next to
the bed, so it will stay charged and ready as a back up in the
event of a power outage.

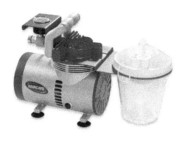
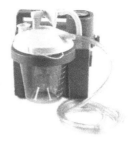

Stationary   Portable

Does Medicare cover two portables instead of one stationary and one portable?

No, you would have to rent or buy an extra portable, but it may be advisable to have an extra one as a reliable backup, especially if you live in an area with frequent power outages. An extra portable machine, with a charged on-board battery is a true backup.

What about the stationary machine?

If you obtain a second portable, keep the Medicare provided stationary machine as a back up in case one of the portable machines needs repair.

What should I ask about suctioning techniques and cleanliness?

Ask a nurse to explain and demonstrate suctioning and then you should demonstrate to the nurse you are able to perform the procedure with an understanding of established protocols (rules) for suctioning techniques and precautions.

At home, ask the technician setting up the equipment about procedures and schedules for cleaning the home healthcare suction machines and changing their related disposables.

Oral suctioning
A rigid suction wand called a Yankauer (below) is used to clear the mouth and is rinsed in tap water between suctioning.

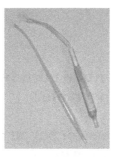

Suction Wands (Yankauers)

Tracheostomy and lung suctioning
A sterile catheter (a thin, flexible, plastic tube) is introduced through the tracheostomy (a surgically created hole in the throat to allow air to pass) into the lungs and is discarded after suctioning.

Consider keeping both machines ready
If your loved one has a tracheostomy, you can keep two bedside home suction machines ready for suctioning. One machine can be set up with an attached rigid suction wand called a Yankauer (above) for the mouth, while the other machine can use an attached sterile flexible catheter for the lungs.

If your loved one needs both the mouth and lungs cleared, you won't have to stop one machine and change attachments from a Yankauer wand to a catheter tube and back. You can use either machine without regard to a set sequence.

<u>Sterile Saline</u>

What is sterile saline solution and does Medicare cover it?

It is sterile salt water and is used, for example, to rinse a sterile catheter during lung suctioning. With a prescription, Medicare covers enough solution needed per day. Your local pharmacy can get and deliver cases of 12, one-liter bottles.

Does the doctor have to write a prescription for each saline delivery?

A six-month standing order will keep the pharmacy from having to request a new prescription every time you need a delivery of saline. Ask the pharmacy what the prescription needs to say, for example, "standing order: six months" or if it needs to state a specified number of refills.

What can I do to make sure I don't run out?

Know the average rate of use per day and watch your supply as it is used up. If a case per month is not enough, ask the doctor to prescribe an additional case per month.

How do I make sure my pharmacy doesn't run out?

Ask your pharmacy to keep an extra case of saline on hand with your loved one's name on it. If you have a standing order, this shouldn't be a burden for the pharmacy. The extra case won't need to be delivered to your loved one sooner than the coverage specifies and you will be protected from it being out of stock. If the pharmacy runs out of saline without an extra case on hand and can't deliver another case on schedule, you'll have to scramble to find another pharmacy with saline in inventory. You'll also have to call the doctor to write an extra prescription for the other pharmacy.

<u>Suction Machine Troubleshooting</u>

The suction is weak.

Check the power connections to the unit, the airflow connections, the air filter and the catch jar. The following tips can be used to troubleshoot machines of most brands.

Stationary
The stationary unit (below left) power cord is hard wired into the machine, so the only power connection to check is at the outlet. If power is not getting to the stationary unit, the stationary machine will not operate.

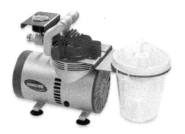
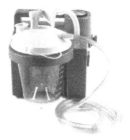

Stationary   Portable

Portable
Has there been enough continuous power to the portable unit (above right) to keep the on-board battery charged? If not and if outlet power is still not getting to the unit, the unit may not work, because the battery is low or dead. If it does operate, it may be with weak suction from a low battery. Starting at the wall outlet and working toward the machine,

the portable unit may have as many as three power connections:

The power cord to the wall outlet
It needs to be firmly plugged into a working wall outlet.

The power cord section from wall to transformer box
There is usually a small transformer box somewhere along the power cord leading to the portable machine. The end of the power cord (opposite the end with the wall outlet plug) needs to be firmly plugged into the transformer box. If the box lies on the floor and it gets kicked or bumped, it may loosen the power connection.

The power cord section from transformer box to machine
It runs to the machine and needs to be firmly plugged into the socket on the side of the machine case. It can vibrate loose, so keep an eye on it.

How can I tell if the power connection to the portable machine is lost?

Many portable machines have a power indicator light on the top of the machine to let you know if there is no power from the wall outlet to the unit. If the light shows this and the machine still runs, it's running off the battery, but the battery is not being charged.

What's an obvious sign the portable unit has not been getting power from the outlet for some time?

If it's been running off the battery and the battery begins to be depleted, the pitch of the suction motor will become lower than usual, because the suction pump motor is running at a slower speed. If you restore outlet power while the pump motor is running, you should hear an immediate change from a lower to a higher (normal) pitch.

The portable machine doesn't run strong from the battery.

After many charge cycles, the on-board battery won't hold a charge very long and needs replacing. If the unit has been charging and runs fine while plugged in, but when you pull the power cord while it is running and it slows way down, the battery may failing.

The unit seems to be running fine and the pitch sounds normal, but the suction is weak.

Check the airflow connections
Are all the plastic air tubes connected and snug? They can look tight, but be a little loose and leak air, reducing suction. Are the air tubes fully connected at both ends of the air filter?

Replace the paper air filter
This is not usually the problem, but suction can be reduced if the paper filter (page 158) gets wet. A wet filter won't pass air and must be replaced, so keep the fluid level from suctioning no higher than 2/3 the way to the top of the catch jar (below). If the filter is old and dirty, replace it.

Check the catch jar and top
Is the catch jar top seated properly on the jar with a good air seal? Look around the edges for anything preventing the alignment between the catch jar and its top. If you hear a loud "pop" after starting the machine, the top wasn't seated on the jar and now it is.

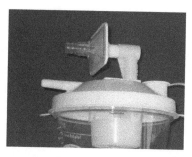

Suction Machine Catch Jar And Top

Maybe the machine pump is getting old
Eventually the suction pump will become weak and will not deliver the same level of suction. If power from the outlet is there and all the air connections and filters check out, the machine is getting tired and needs repair or replacement.

Is there a quick way to check the pump strength and locate an air leak?

Shut the machine off and pull the air suction tube from the machine case. Turn it on and put your thumb over the hole on the machine case where the tube was connected. If the suction is strong, the suction pump is not the problem. If the suction is weak and the portable machine is plugged into a working wall outlet, the pump is the problem. You need to repair or replace the machine.

If the pump is working properly, you can use the same test to find an air leak. Moving outward from the machine case where you did the test mentioned above, reconnect each tube section and test it. As each section checks out, connect the next piece and test the end of it. When the suction feels weak, you'll know the air leak is in the section of tubing you just connected.

What about spare suction machine air filters?

Ask the technician from the home healthcare company for spare paper air filters. The stationary machine has a different air filter (below left) than the portable air filter (below right). Change the air filter if it gets wet or looks dirty.

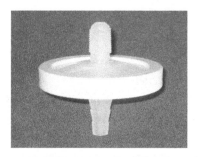 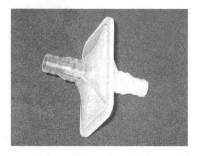

Stationary Air Filter   Portable Air Filter

Chapter 9

Antibiotics And Infection Prevention

The use of antibiotics is an effective treatment to counter infection and can give your loved one a chance to continue to participate in physical therapy to gain strength and stamina and stay on the path to recovery.

Doctors can't examine your loved one daily at home, so they rely on your educated observations and accurate recall of vital information received over the phone. You are a primary communicator calling the doctor with updated information, including the apparent effectiveness of prescribed antibiotics.

Bacterial infections and the use of antibiotics are common in hospitals and at home, so this chapter provides you with a basic familiarity with antibiotics as well as some of their benefits and hazards. A basic understanding of antibiotics can help you make a positive difference in the home healthcare of your loved one, especially if the infections are repeating or are chronic (long-term).

What are antibiotics?

Antibiotics are given to kill or weaken bacteria. Since they only treat bacterial infections, they are useless against viral and fungal infections and each antibiotic is effective only for certain types of bacterial infections. If there is an allergy to an antibiotic, it can eliminate the class of antibiotic from consideration. Your doctor will also take into account common side effects.

Why should I care about understanding antibiotics?

The most suitable antibiotic taken as directed can allow those who are weak and sickly after a hospital stay to gain strength, engage in physical therapy and stay well long enough to get better. If you know about common problems with antibiotics, you can play a valuable part observing your loved one and communicating with the doctor to make sure your loved one stays on the path toward healing and recovery.

Problems With Antibiotics

What kinds of problems can there be with antibiotics?

The wrong one
If the antibiotic is not the right one for the infection, it will not get rid of it. If the symptoms do not start to go away in a few days, call the doctor who will assess the suitability of the antibiotic.

Resistance
If an antibiotic has been working well for repeating

infections, but is losing its effectiveness, it will no longer completely get rid of the infection. If the symptoms do not go away as fast as they did with the same previous infections, mention it to the doctor who will decide if the antibiotic should have a substitute. He may decide to alternate equally effective antibiotics to delay the infectious bacteria from adapting to either one. To prevent resistance, here are some guidelines:

- Take as directed and take the full course (prescribed duration) of an antibiotic even if the symptoms are gone.
- Stay in touch with the doctor as to how well the antibiotic is working.
- To battle repeating infections, ask the doctor about alternating antibiotics (page 167) from infection to infection.

More powerful than needed
An antibiotic may work well, but it may be so powerful it takes away all your loved one's physical energy, so the infection will go away, but during the course (prescribed duration) of the antibiotic, your loved one will be lying in bed losing muscle strength and stamina. To maintain as much energy as possible for physical therapy, the antibiotic should be no stronger than necessary. Ask the doctor if there is a less powerful, but effective one available.

Harm to the body
Another reason the antibiotic should be no stronger than necessary is the more powerful the antibiotic, the more harm it does to the body. The kidneys take a hit every time a "blockbuster" antibiotic is given, so use of the most powerful antibiotics is suited for serious infections where no other

antibiotic will work. The most powerful are usually delivered intravenously and for the following reason (cost) as well, such "blockbusters" may not be a long-term solution to treat your loved one's repeating infections.

Cost
Medicare does not cover intravenous (IV) antibiotics given at home. Because they are extremely expensive, ask the doctor if there is an effective antibiotic that can be taken "by mouth" (or crushed and put into the feeding tube) instead. Medicare (and insurance) is likely to cover this type of non-IV antibiotic given at home.

If an IV antibiotic is necessary and, like most people, you can't afford it, ask the doctor if your loved one can visit the hospital each day for the IV antibiotic to be given on an outpatient basis or can be readmitted to the hospital for the duration of the antibiotic.

Allergic reactions
Antibiotics can cause allergic reactions. If a reaction occurs, even if it's from an antibiotic (or any medicine) taken successfully in the past, call the doctor. Stay observant, because minor allergic reactions can develop into major ones. Ask the doctor what to look for.

Thinning of the blood
If your loved one is also on a blood thinner, your doctor may order extra blood clotting analyses during the course (prescribed duration) of an antibiotic. If the blood gets too thin, he may restrict exercise activity, because of the potential for internal bleeding. Once the laboratory report shows the blood is again thick enough (due to an adjustment of blood thinning medicine doses and/or naturally after

the end of the antibiotic course), he may allow exercise to resume.

Interference by other medicines
Go over your loved one's medicines list and ask the doctor if a regularly taken medicine can negatively affect the absorption or effectiveness of the antibiotic. The fine print on the information sheet included with an antibiotic may warn against giving specific medicines too close in time to giving the antibiotic. Ask the doctor how to schedule the antibiotic doses.

Side effects
If you see anything different about your loved one after an antibiotic is started, call the doctor. Side effects are common and some are acceptable to the doctor and while others are not. Call the doctor to report, for example: stomachache, queasiness or nausea. The doctor may substitute another antibiotic.

A common side effect is diarrhea. It's not only embarrassing and uncomfortable, but it can dehydrate your loved one and cause rashes, sores and bladder infections. If your loved one is tube fed (Chapter 10), ask the doctor about preventing diarrhea by changing the feeding formula before the first dose for the duration of the antibiotic (page 182) and preventing constipation by changing the formula back to normal after the antibiotic course (prescribed duration) is complete.

Yeast infections
Naturally occurring yeast in the body is kept in check by friendly bacteria. Antibiotics reduce the good bacteria, so yeast may multiply enough to cause, for example a vaginal yeast infection or a yeast infection of the mouth, called

Thrush. Ask the doctor about prevention and treatment.

Additional issues
Ask the doctor to review these and other potential antibiotic issues and explain how they relate to your loved one's medical condition and treatment.

Antibiotics At Home

How can I help manage the antibiotics?

Now that your loved one is home trying to recover strength and stamina, you are the primary observer. If you learn from the doctor what to watch for in terms of infection onset and understand the benefits and limitations of antibiotics, you will do much to help the doctor optimize the care and recovery at home.

How can I learn of an antibiotic's potential allergies and side effects?

Ask the doctor at the time she mentions the antibiotic. You can ask the pharmacist and read the information sheet with the container. Here is a great resource:

http://www.drugs.com/

My loved one has queasiness from an antibiotic.

Empty stomach or full?
Some antibiotics cause digestive problems if given when your loved one has an empty stomach or after the tube feeding has been interrupted. Ask the doctor about the antibiotic and how it should be given, because taking antibiotics incorrectly may also reduce or eliminate effectiveness.

Maybe the antibiotic was not the primary cause after all
Some people need to be quiet for at least an hour before and after taking medicines like potassium liquid, which can cause queasiness and nausea. The better you observe, the more you can help the doctor.

Surrounding circumstances
Was anything different when you gave the antibiotic this time? Did the usual exercise, feeding or giving medicines time change relative to the antibiotic time?

Minor Digestive Problem Remedies

What about minor digestive problems that don't occur during the use of an antibiotic?

Ask the doctor for an opinion before trying anything on your own. She might recommend a common over the counter remedy or prescribe a medicine.

Why should I bother the doctor about a digestive problem that doesn't seem serious?

Don't assume it isn't serious or can't become so. The wrong remedy or medicine can make a minor problem worse. If you ask family, friends or if you have visiting nurses, you may hear varying opinions. Let the doctor diagnose and settle it.

Starting An Antibiotic

What is there to consider when starting an antibiotic?

It is helpful to try a "new" (new to the patient) antibiotic or other "new" medicine on a day your doctor is reachable, so if there is a problem, you can discuss it with your doctor.

Due to feeding, exercise and medicine schedules, there are better times than others to give an antibiotic. Ask the doctor what times are best for your loved one's daily routine.

The antibiotic arrived at 4 P.M., but the best dosing times are 9 P.M. and 9 A.M. What are our options to get on the dosing schedule?

Ask the doctor about three options:

Waiting
Should you wait five more hours until 9 P.M. to give the 1st dose? You'll be on schedule, but the sooner the antibiotic is given, the sooner the infection will start to go away.

Giving it right away
If you need to be on a schedule like 9 P.M. and 9 A.M., you could give the 1st dose right away at 4 P.M. and give the 2nd dose at 9 P.M. This would be only five hours later, instead of the ordered 12 hours between doses, so ask the doctor if it is O.K. You may not want to do this if you are concerned about more antibiotic than necessary in the stomach. It might amplify some side effects of the antibiotic, resulting in a higher risk for queasiness, nausea and diarrhea.

Staggering the doses
You could give the 1st dose right away at 4 P.M., give the 2nd dose at 2 A.M. (10 hrs later), the 3rd at 12 noon the next day (10 hrs later), the 4th dose the next evening at 9 P.M. (9 hrs later) and the 5th dose at 9 A.M. (12 hrs later) the following morning. This method will gradually achieve the 9 P.M. and 9 A.M. schedule. Ask the doctor what times to give the initial doses to "ramp in" to the preferred schedule.

166

<u>Alternating Antibiotics</u>

Why does the doctor need to alternate antibiotics from infection to infection and what is my role?

The purpose is to delay as long as possible the bacteria causing repeating infections from adapting to the antibiotic. Tell the doctor if you think an antibiotic seems to be losing its effectiveness, so the doctor can decide to have it discontinued and introduce a new antibiotic into the rotation.

With longer-term antibiotics, resistance is inevitable and the doctor may not remember the same antibiotic is still being given, so stay observant and don't wait for the doctor to ask if it is still working. Use your journal to track how long the same antibiotics have been used, because you will eventually begin to see reduced effectiveness of either or both.

A certain antibiotic started producing mild allergic reactions, so it was discontinued. Can it ever be used again?

Maybe. The catch is an allergic reaction test must be done every time. Doctors start with a minute amount and increase it with each dose and if they reach the required dose with no reaction, they might continue it. The problem is the initial test is not a predictor of an allergic reaction if the same antibiotic is given for the next infection, so the next time they consider prescribing it, they must conduct the same test again. The test is not usually performed unless other practical alternatives to the antibiotic have been exhausted.

Why do doctors prefer to wait for symptoms to become more pronounced before allowing an antibiotic?

Waiting for symptoms to be pronounced helps diagnose the infection and allows the immune system to fight the infection with an acceptable fever. Elevated body temperature is a natural defense mechanism to inhibit infectious bacterial growth. Overuse of antibiotics is a concern, so giving antibiotics later in the onset of infection may help delay the infectious bacteria in developing antibiotic resistance. Starting the antibiotic later also means a shorter course (prescribed duration), which lessens the antibiotic's toll on the body, especially the kidneys.

Chronic, Repeating Infections And Antibiotics

My loved one seems stuck in a never-ending cycle of repeating bacterial infections sapping her energy and preventing her from exercising often enough to gain strength and stamina. What can I do?

Infections may cause your loved one days of lethargy while you wait for symptoms to intensify enough to justify giving an antibiotic. Each day your loved one is not moving forward with exercise, she is losing strength and stamina. If a specific and sustained fever level is needed to allow the antibiotic, it may occur days after the beginning of decreased energy, an inability to exercise and other familiar symptoms of infection.

Ask the doctor about changing the decision to start an antibiotic, because if the decision is based less on the fever level and more upon all symptoms, it may allow you to call the doctor for an antibiotic approval earlier in the onset of an infection. The sooner you start the antibiotic, the fewer exercise days lost to lethargy. Your loved one may recover and resume exercise sooner, which builds strength.

Will my doctor be receptive to an idea like this?

You won't know if you don't ask. If your doctor trusts your observations when you call to report symptoms and has a common sense attitude about being flexible and creative, there is a good chance you will be allowed to try this kind of earlier intervention.

What can I hope to see as my loved one improves?

Your loved one may became stronger, happier, healthier and better at fighting off infections, making the symptoms milder and shorter-lived. The average interval between infections may become longer. If so, the number of days with exercising will increase, allowing for more improvement.

What kinds of infections interfere with recovery?

Repeat bacterial infections of the lungs and bladder are among those that can interfere with the recovery progress, especially if your loved one is elderly.

What are some common symptoms of these infections?

Lung infections symptoms include: bad breath or a foul odor coming from the tracheostomy (a surgically created hole in the throat to allow air to pass), lethargy, weakness, shorter lived episodes of fever becoming elevated and longer lasting, thickening and darkening mucus and chest congestion. Ask the doctor to list and explain all your loved one's symptoms.

Bladder infection symptoms include, bad smelling urine, a change in urine color, pain in the bladder, fever, lethargy and weakness. Ask the doctor to list and explain all your loved one's symptoms.

How can I tell as early as possible if my loved one has an infection?

There are typical symptoms, but your loved one may or may not be typical of a person with an infection. There may or may not be a change in behavior (other than fatigue) and there may be no mental confusion (even if elderly), which is part of what doctors and nurses watch for during an infection onset.

Ask the doctor to list the standard symptoms to watch for and note in them your journal as well as the symptoms your loved one exhibits with each infection and the name of each infection the doctor diagnoses. If your loved one has repeating infections, you will become familiar with the early onset symptoms.

What should I keep in mind?

It's not about using antibiotics to knock out infection after infection while your loved one gets weaker and weaker. It's about handling the infections in a subjective way using common sense. The goal is to have your loved one bounce back sooner to participate in exercise and stay well long enough to get better.

<u>Antibiotic Measures To Keep Infections Away</u>

My loved one has repeating lung and bladder infections. Do doctors ever give antibiotics to prevent or delay infections?

Ask about standing orders of antibiotics to keep certain repeating infections away. Actually, this doesn't prevent infection, but it may reduce the frequency, severity and duration of symptoms.

For example, an antibiotic aerosol mist may be inhaled for lung infections (next topic) and a dilute antibiotic solution may be given via a disposable sterile urethral catheter into the bladder for bladder infections (page 173).

<u>Lung Infection Treatment With A Nebulizer</u>

What is a compressor/nebulizer device?

A specialized compressor (below left) forces air through a tube to an attached disposable nebulizer (below right), which holds and atomizes the liquid dose of medicine. From the nebulizer, the medicine is delivered via an attached air hose as a wet aerosol (a mist to be inhaled).

Asthma medicines are commonly nebulized and inhaled. Some antibiotics can be inhaled for certain lung infections. This method may be effective for a lung infection well under way or it may be effective as a long-term therapy to delay infection.

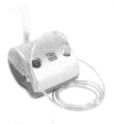 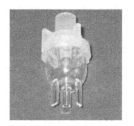

Compressor   Nebulizer

If your doctor wants your loved one to use a nebulizer to deliver a medicine, ask a nurse to train you to set it up and get the medicine mist properly flowing.

Does Medicare cover this type of machine?

In some cases, so ask the doctor about inhaled medicines. Medicare covers the compressor as capped rental equipment for 13 continuous months and then it's given to your loved one. The disposables are covered as well.

Bladder Infection Prevention

What can be done to reduce the frequency, severity and duration of repeating bacterial bladder infections?

A urologist (a doctor who focuses on the urinary tracts of males and females and on the reproductive system of males) may recommend the following:

One: Remove the Foley catheter
If the bladder doesn't empty enough each time, urine left behind can create a haven for bacteria to proliferate and cause an infection. A urethral catheter and drain bag called a Foley (below) is used at the hospital to keep the bladder

empty and measure urine output. It is usually changed only about once a month, so as a long-term, invasive medical device, the urethral catheter can act as a conduit for bacteria to enter the bladder.

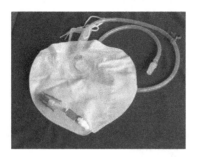

Foley

Two: Use intermittent catheterizing to empty the bladder
Intermittent catheterizing is an effective alternative to a Foley catheter. Instead of the Foley catheter, empty the bladder as often as directed with a disposable sterile urethral catheter and attached drain bag. This procedure can introduce bacteria, but it may work better to reduce infections than leaving a Foley catheter in place or doing nothing at all. For more information:

http://www.nlm.nih.gov/medlineplus/ency/article/003972.htm

What are the challenges of intermittent catheterizing?

Skin irritation
Regularly inserting and removing a urethral catheter may irritate urethral tissues. Ask the nurses at the hospital about this issue and what you can do to minimize and treat it.

Accuracy of measurement
With disposable catheters and drain bags, the bag volume
markings are not consistent from bag to bag, so you need
to pour the collected urine into a measuring cup and then
record the date, time and quantity on a chart for "liquids
out". If you measure "liquids in" (page 39), also measure
"liquids out".

Three: Push a dilute antibiotic rinse into the bladder
A dilute antibiotic solution can be delivered via a disposible
sterile catheter into the bladder. This practice helps protect
the bladder against bacteria, including any introduced by the
intermittent catheterizing.

For procedures at home requiring a urethral catheter, ask the
nurses at the hospital for training before your loved one is
discharged.

Four: Add daily cranberry juice to the water intake
Cranberry juice has an inhibitive effect on bladder infections,
which may help reduce the frequency of symptoms.

What should I know about cranberry juice?

Sugar content
At the store, examine the content labels for sugar, because
some brands are much higher in sugar than others.
"Unsweetened" has lower sugar, so start there.

Acidity
Fruit juice is higher in acidity than water, so if your loved
one is taking an antacid to reduce stomach acidity, you may
need to find a substitute for the juice. Try CranActin, a liquid
cranberry syrup extract (below). A few drops mixed with
water may provide a good substitute without the sugar and

acidity. Keep it refrigerated. It's at natural foods stores, but you can save by buying from an Internet vendor like VitaNet.

http://www.vitanetonline.com/

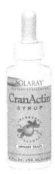

CranActin Syrup (2 oz.)
Copyright 2009 NutraMarks, Inc.

What if my loved one is being fed through a tube?

You can add the drops of the syrup to regular infusions of water pushed into the stomach tube (for adequate hydration) or add it to the formula in the feeding bag. Dried, crushed and grinded cranberry skins are also available at natural food stores, but they are likely to clog the feeding tube.

General Cleanliness And Infection Prevention Measures

How can I help keep germs down and prevent infections?

This is an important issue, so these measures are essential, especially if your loved one is still weakened from illness or is elderly.

Hand washing
Require all who visit the residence to stop at the kitchen sink and wash their hands, so it is done before they enter the bedroom. Use paper towels, because cloth towels harbor germs.

Sanitizer gels
In addition to all other infection prevention measures, frequently use hand sanitizer gels. Make sure you keep the dispensers out of the reach of children and pets, because they like to taste attractively scented gels, which can cause alcohol toxicity.

Using gloves
Gloves can be effective for the bedside caregiver, but change them often, because as soon as the gloves touch a surface, they start picking up germs. Gloves not changed often enough will protect the hands of the wearer, not your loved one.

Disinfecting the bedroom and bathroom
Put on gloves and use a disinfectant to wipe down frequently touched surfaces like doorknobs and bed rails. Clean the toilet, countertops and sinks of the your loved one's bathroom at least twice a week. The more often it is done, the better. If you hire a caregiver, cleaning the bedroom and the bathroom is part of her job. The rest of the residence is not.

Eye precautions
Try to prevent your loved one from putting her fingers into her eyes. Using fingers to rub the eyes causes eye infections and transmits colds. Rubbing can also scratch eye surfaces, especially if fingernails are long or sharp. Use an emery board regularly to file the nails down to the fingertips.

Fingernail precautions
Germs can enter the bloodstream via tiny cuts in the skin, so don't trim fingernails too close and leave the cuticles alone. If you trim the nails with clippers, err on leaving too much nail and use an emery board to sand them the rest of the way down.

Toenail precautions
Due to the risk of infection to those weakened by illness, don't let anyone except a podiatrist trim and cut toenails. Medicare pays for periodic home visits by a podiatrist to a "homebound" (leaving the home requires considerable and taxing effort) person.

If a toenail needs shortening before the next covered visit by the podiatrist, use an emery board. If there is a sharp nail edge irritating another toe, emery it down. A footbath with Epsom salts works very well to keep the skin of the toes and toenails healthy. Ask the doctor if this is O.K.

Chapter 10

Tube Feeding Issues And Tips

This chapter reviews common tube feeding issues and offers tips, so your daily experience with tube feeding, the formulas and feeding equipment will go as smoothly as possible.

Tube feeding is not difficult to understand or perform. You can do this!

If tube feeding will be continued at home, ask to be trained by nurses at the hospital in daily tube feeding methods, nutritional requirements, giving supplemental water via the feeding tube, infection prevention precautions and equipment troubleshooting techniques.

Topics here include a basic orientation with tube feeding, the formulas, formula attributes and selection criteria, changing the formula during an antibiotic, Medicare coverage and feeding tube replacement issues. There are also tips on setting up and troubleshooting the feeding equipment and clearing occasional clogs in the feeding tube.

Tube Feeding Basics

What do I need to know about tube feeding?

The right formula or mixture of formulas
Your loved one needs appropriate nutrition, adequate daily calories and a formula or mixture of formulas to maintain correct stool consistency, so there is neither constipation nor diarrhea.

The rate of flow, duration and feeding times
Discuss these considerations with your loved one's doctor and dietician. The rate should be high enough to deliver an adequate volume of prescribed formula per day, the duration of flow should continue for medicines that need to be taken on a full or partially full stomach and the timing should allow for interruptions for bedside caregiving tasks, therapy and to give the digestive tract a rest.

Regularly flushing the feeding tube
If formula or medicines are left too long in the tube and begin to crystallize, the feeding tube can clog. The age of the tube (usually six to nine months) will eventually create increasing episodes of clogging until it is replaced. No matter how old the tube, a clog can be difficult to clear and if it cannot be resolved quickly enough to resume feeding, water infusions and medicines, it may need to be replaced.

Ask a nurse to explain how, how often and before and after which daily events the tube should be flushed to keep it clear. Because plain water (in addition to feeding formula) is regularly infused daily into the stomach to assure proper hydration, use water to flush the tube.

Cleanliness
Always thoroughly wash your hands before you set up a new disposable feeding bag with the feeding pump and before you fill a new bag with formula. The bag should be changed at least once every 24 hours, but ask the doctor how often. Don't reuse bags. Don't keep adding formula to the bag beyond the recommended time limit or it can spoil in the bag. Flush the stomach tube regularly to prevent clogs and so formula won't remain in the stomach tube where it can spoil and cause diarrhea. Ask the technician setting up the equipment how to keep the pump clean.

Expiration dates
Be sure to mark the expiration dates of the formula on the outside of each case in large bold ink. Store the formula as directed, so it won't spoil before it expires.

Can I get a quick lesson in the formulas?

Tube feeding formulas are pre-mixed and referred to as enteral formulas. There are three attributes to consider when choosing a formula:

- Nutritional (including mineral and fiber) content
- Caloric content
- Osmolality

Each nutritional attribute is expressed on the label in a "per ml" or "per cc" format. (1 ml. = 1 cc.) (240 ml. = 1 cup)

Nutritional content
Formulas are designed to give adequate nutrition, while varying to conform to the medical conditions of patients. There are formulas lower in sodium and lower or higher in fiber. Some are higher in protein and calories, so a lower

volume of formula can still deliver enough calories per day when a lower infusion (pump) rate must be used.

Caloric content
This is a familiar term used to describe food energy content. The doctor and dietician will recommend a formula and volume per day to meet your loved one's daily requirement.

Osmolality
Each pre-mixed formula has an osmolality number you can find on the container. A higher osmolality number indicates a formula making the stool softer than a formula with a lower number.

I'm not a dietician, so why should I care about what's in the formula?

To get the osmolality right
To give optimal osmolality, not too low or too high, your loved one may need a regular daily formula of a specific osmolality or a mixture of two formulas with one having a higher and the other a lower osmolality. Each person and medical condition is unique, so there will be some trial and error (loose or hard stools) before you get the best formula or mixture of two formulas set for your loved one.

To make a temporary change for antibiotics
Each formula has a tendency (shown by its osmolality number on the container) to cause constipation or diarrhea. Antibiotics also have a tendency to cause diarrhea. To head off diarrhea during a course (prescribed duration) of antibiotic, try temporarily changing to a formula with a lower osmolality number until the antibiotic treatment ends.

To change back after antibiotics end
After the last day of an antibiotic, you will need to change back to the higher osmolality formula or mixture of two formulas to prevent constipation.

To make changes to adapt to your loved one
Over time, as your loved one gets better and stronger or gains weight, the formulas may have to change. If you need advice about other formulas, speak with the doctor, the dietician who recommended the original formulas and the pharmacist who fills the formula prescription.

The maker may discontinue your formula
If this happens, go to their website to see the recommended substitute. Be sure to check all three attributes, so you can be sure it is a good fit for your loved one's needs. Also, check the sodium content. You can call the company supplying the tube feeding and speak with their pharmacist. You can also call the supervising dietician at the hospital where your loved one stayed. As with all decisions, clear it with the doctor.

How can I find the best mix of formulas for regular feeding?

Temporary constipation is preferable to diarrhea, so start with a doctor/dietician-approved formula with the lowest osmolality number. If the stools are too hard, adjust the feeding by substituting a container of the lower numbered formula with a container of the higher numbered formula. When stools reach the correct softness, the ratio of the formula mixture for regular feeding is set.

How can I obtain two different formulas to make temporary formula mixture changes?

When you discuss the formula prescription with the doctor, ask her to order two formulas, one with the highest and the other with the lowest possible osmolality numbers appropriate for your loved one. You can mix the formulas to keep the right stool consistency. When antibiotics are needed, change the mixture toward the lower numbered formula to prevent diarrhea. When the antibiotics are over, change toward the higher numbered formula to prevent constipation.

How can I ensure the temporary formula change will be made?

Post a memo with large print near the bed to tell everyone the date the formula is being changed and until what date. Also, remove from the room the containers of formula you don't want used.

For additional information on the basics of tube feeding:

http://www.csun.edu/~cjh78264/tubefeeding/index.html

Tube Feeding Equipment And Formula Coverage

What is needed for tube feeding Medicare coverage?

You need a prescription stating the medical reason for tube feeding, the specific feeding formula(s) and the number of cans or bottles (fluid volume) consumed per 24-hour day.

What does Medicare cover for tube feeding?

Medicare covers the intravenous (IV) pole, the tube feeding pump and monthly supplies of premixed formulas and disposable feeding bags.

IV pole
The pole supports an attached feeding pump and has upper arms to support a suspended feeding bag. Intravenous medication bags can also be suspended from the pole arms.

Tube feeding pump
There are many pumps and models from various manufacturers. The home healthcare company should train you at home when they deliver the system and set it up. The pump plugs into the house current and usually, there is an on-board rechargeable battery to power the pump in the event of a power failure.

Supplies of formula
Your loved one's doctor, typically after consulting with a dietician, will approve which formula or combination of formulas is most suitable and how much volume per day is needed.

Tube Feeding Clog Prevention And Clearing Tips

The feeding tube to the stomach keeps getting clogged.

As formula passes through the feeding tube, its protein, sugars and fiber can crystallize and coat the inside of the tube. To prevent clogging, you need to regularly flush the tube with water to rinse it clean. Flushing after giving medicines via the tube is important, so ask a nurse how often and when to regularly flush the tube.

Do you have specific clog prevention tips?

Liquids other than water can interact with medicines
Ask nurses about your loved one's medicines. For example, using Coca-Cola to flush the tube after giving an antacid may cause the residual antacid in the tube to form sticky clumps and clog the tube.

Flush between each medicine
Medicine still in the tube can react with the next one to cause a clog. Ask a nurse which medicines in combination are likely to do this.

No solids in the tube
Don't put anything fibrous down the tube. If fiber is part of a pre-mixed feeding formula, it's O.K., but flush the tube as directed by the nurse.

Fully pulverize pills first
If you give pills via the tube, you have to fully crush them first. You can buy a pill crusher at the local pharmacy. Some medicines are time-release and should never be crushed, so ask the doctor or pharmacist. Crush the medicine until powdered and mix it in a solution of warm water. After you give the medicine, flush the tube with more water.

What should I use to flush the tube?

Use water, because it is chemically neutral and is needed throughout the day as part of nutrition. If the formula in the feeding tube begins to slow down and water is not doing the trick to dissolve clogs, try Diet Caffeine Free Coke, because it has no sugar, caffeine or high acidity. Cranberry juice or Regular Coke will work, but both contain a lot of sugar. Natural (unsweetened and filtered) cranberry juice works, but it has the higher acidity of fruit juice.

How often should I flush the tube?

Every time the feeding bag tube is either disconnected or reconnected to the stomach feeding tube, flush the stomach feeding tube. If the feeding bag runs out of formula, flush the tube before you either stopper the tube or connect another bag of formula. If you give medicine through the stomach tube, flush it before and after, so the entire dose of the medicine goes into the stomach and the medicine won't remain in the stomach tube to interact with feeding formula in the tube to form a clog.

What should I try if the formula stops flowing through the stomach feeding tube?

The tube may not be clogged. Try changing the body position, because the tube could be kinked inside the body and the change could free it up.

The stomach tube is clogged, so what can I do?

Use a 60 cc catheter tip syringe (below) to pull residual fluid out of the tube. Then fill the syringe with and push a clog-dissolving liquid into the tube. Try Diet Caffeine Free Coke, because it is bubbly and dissolves most clogs. For more stubborn clogs, try super bubbly water, like Perrier. It is extremely carbonated, so it may work if Coke doesn't.

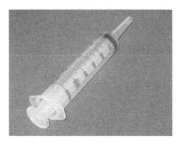

60 cc Catheter Tip Syringe

If a clog is very stubborn, what else can I do?

After pulling out the liquids already tried, put a little warm water into the syringe, push it into the clogged tube and let it sit in the tube for a few minutes. After it cools, use the syringe to replace the cool water with another batch of warm water. Then pump the syringe plunger GENTLY in very rapid, firm and short pulses (like a mini-jackhammer). The heat and vibration may clear the worst clogs.

It's still clogged. What now?

Leave some Diet Caffeine Free Coke or Perrier in the tube for a few hours or overnight and do the previously mentioned procedures again. Time can be the secret ingredient for unclogging a tube.

We've tried everything, but the tube is still clogged.

If the feeding tube becomes clogged and you can't clear it, you may have to take your loved one to the hospital and have the tube replaced. Due to wear and tear, it will have to be replaced about every six to nine months, but a stubborn clog may cause it to be replaced sooner.

Feeding Tube Replacement

Why are clogs happening more often and becoming more stubborn?

If the tube is six to nine months old, it could be getting old. The end of the tube could be clogging and collapsing from long-term exposure to digestive acids. As the inside of the tube opening in the digestive tract deteriorates, it becomes more vulnerable to clogging from buildup of formula and medicines.

How urgent it is to get the tube replaced?

It depends
The urgency depends on how long the tube has been clogged and what the clog is preventing your loved one from receiving (water, medicines, formula). It also depends upon the presence of a second tube to use while trying to unclog the blocked tube. If a second tube is not present, you need to consider how long it will take to replace the clogged tube with a new one.

If there is only one tube
If you have only one tube and it is clogged and you can't clear it within a short time, call the doctor and ask how much time flexibility there is for an interruption in water, medicines and feeding, while you keep trying to clear the tube.

If attempts to clear the tube aren't working, a decision has to be made far enough in advance to have the tube replacement scheduled and performed at the hospital.

If it is a dual (two) tube system
If you have two tubes and only one is clogged, the doctor

might give you more time to try to clear the clog before you have to decide to arrange for a tube replacement procedure.

If there is one tube to the stomach and another tube to the small intestine, so as long as one of the tubes is working, replacement is not as urgent. If the tube can't be cleared, the tube system should be replaced as soon as possible, so each tube can be used for its intended purpose and in case the remaining working tube stops working or becomes clogged.

Are two tubes better than one?

When your loved one is at the hospital to get the feeding tube system for the first time, ask your doctor to order a dual (two) tube system. If one of the tubes clogs, you'll have the other to use, while you try to unclog the blocked tube. If two tubes were ordered, verify the order by looking at the top of the tube system for two ports (openings) with the letters: G and J.

How routine is the tube system replacement procedure?

The tube system is replaced about every six to nine months. The surgeon uses the same opening in the abdominal wall and follows the same pathways into the stomach and into the small intestine for each replacement. Try to schedule it for mid-morning, so your loved may be home by late afternoon.

Feeding Pump Issues

What should I ask about the feeding pump?

The technician/trainer needs to do more than show you how to set up the equipment. Ask him to describe and demonstrate common problems and show you how to solve them. Take notes and put them in your journal. Ask for the technical support phone number and the after hours number and tape the numbers on the pump. Before he leaves, make sure you know how to:

- Set the digital touch panel flow rate and volume per day
- Reset the rate and volume settings
- Set up and get the liquid formula flowing
- Troubleshoot common problems

The feeding pump is broken and needs replacing.

A broken pump is a fairly rare occurrence, but you should know what you can do to make the replacement proceed smoothly. Tell the technician you want the replacement pump to be the same brand and model, so you don't have to be retrained on the new machine. Feeding bags work with a specific pump brand, so your supply might not work if the new pump is not the same brand as the old one. If they have to bring a pump that uses different bags, remind the supplier to bring a case (one month supply) of the feeding bags specified for the new pump.

Feeding Bag Issues

What about tube feeding bags?

Medicare covers deliveries of monthly supplies of tube feeding formula and feeding bags. When you call the supplier for the monthly formula delivery, remind them not to forget the bags and restate the type of bag your pump uses. If you don't, the supplier could forget to bring the bags or deliver the wrong type. While the delivery person is still at the residence, make sure the bags are right for your pump.

Where should I get the feeding equipment and formulas?

You can get all needed feeding items from a home healthcare company (page 75) or a specialty pharmacy (page 52). It can be very beneficial to establish a good relationship with a reputable specialty pharmacy. In the event your loved one's nutritional needs change or the formula is discontinued by the manufacturer, a specialty pharmacist's knowledge of a possible substitute formula's contents and purpose can be helpful in selecting the best replacement. Your specialty pharmacist may be more available for a phone consultation than your loved one's hospital stay dietician.

Y Port Tube Feeding Adapter

What other useful tube feeding equipment is there?

A "Y port adapter" (below left) is kept inserted in a feeding tube opening. Like the opening into which it inserts, the adapter's opening can accept a feeding bag tube tip (below center) or a 60 cc catheter tip syringe for infusing water (below right). On the side of the adapter, you can see a small side port. This port is used to infuse medicines without the need to interrupt the feeding pump.

This device is first mentioned on page 45 to remind you to request spares as your loved one is discharged from the hospital. If visiting nurses (page 60) come to the residence, they may be able to supply adapter replacements. Otherwise, see Appendix 5 for ordering more as they wear out. They last about six months.

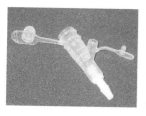 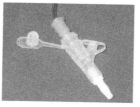 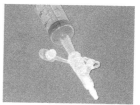

Y Port Adapter   Feeding Bag Tip   Catheter Syringe

There are two feeding tubes, so do I really need a Y port adapter?

If there are two tubes, you may not need an adapter for its intended purpose: to allow uninterrupted feeding while giving medicine through the feeding tube. Even with two tubes, you may find it useful to use one adapter for the following reasons:

The adapter helps prevent tube mix-ups
The G tube (gastric/stomach) and the J tube (jejunal/small intestine) openings look almost identical, so attaching one adapter to either opening makes it much easier to visually distinguish them. Ask the doctor about your loved one's condition and if getting them mixed up could create a medical difficulty and how serious it might be.

The adapter helps extend the life of the tube system
The adapter protects the feeding tube opening and its attached stopper from stretching out or breaking due to repeated use. Once an unprotected feeding tube opening or its stopper wears out, the entire tube system needs replacement at the hospital. When the adapter's opening becomes stretched or the adapter stopper gives out, you can pull out the adapter and insert a new one into the feeding tube opening. The adapter keeps trips to the hospital to replace the tube system as far apart as possible.

There are two tubes, so why not use two adapters to protect both openings?

If you use two adapters, you will protect both the G and J tube openings, but the openings will again look almost exactly alike and you will eventually get them mixed up. If your doctor says you can use either tube, go ahead and use two adapters to protect both tube openings.

If it does matter which tube is used for formula or medicines, then use only one adapter, so you won't get the tube openings confused. Once you decide which opening (the one used most often) to attach the adapter, don't remove it except to replace it and, in doing so, be careful you don't mistakenly change it to the other opening.

Tube Feeding Equipment Troubleshooting

The liquid formula has stopped flowing from the bag.

First, try to flush the stomach tube with water to make sure it is not clogged. If the stomach tube will not flush, it is blocked due to a kink or a clog. If it is clear, check the feeding pump, the feeding bag and the feeding bag tube. If the following tips don't solve the problem, call technical support at the supply company.

Feeding pump
Is there electric power to the pump?
If the power has been off for quite awhile, the pump on-board battery may be depleted and needs recharging.
Is the pump volume/duration setting stopping the formula?
Is the pump flow sensor clean?
Is the formula at the right level in the pump flow sensor bulb?

Feeding bag and tube
Is the feeding bag (below left) out of formula?
Is there an air pocket in the bag tube (below right)?
Is the feeding bag tube kinked? Examine the tube, especially where it exits the bag (below right).

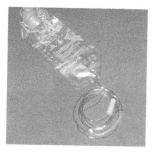

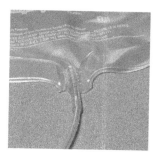

Feeding Bag

Feeding Bag Tube

Chapter 11

Original Medicare, Private Insurance And Billing Issues

I know what you're thinking...

Do I really have to know about Medicare and insurance? I've already got enough to think about. Just send me the bills. How tough could it be?

If your loved one received goods or services from a medical provider such as a hospital, specialty pharmacy or a home healthcare company and you pay the bills without referring to this chapter, you may never know if:

- You were overcharged for the good or service.
- You paid for the same thing twice.
- You were pressed for a payment not yet owed.
- A bill was not really Past Due.
- A bill or a larger part of it might have been covered, had you provided the billing party with additional information.
- You could have appealed the coverage decision.

This chapter also explains communicating with billing departments and avoiding the "run around" with insurance companies.

With a basic understanding of Medicare and insurance, you will know if the bills have properly gone through Medicare and insurance submission and processing to result in amounts your loved one should owe.

<u>Medicare And Insurance Basics</u>

How can you help me with Medicare and insurance?

This chapter will explain basic concepts and show you how to deal with Medicare, insurance companies and providers of medical goods and services.

What topics are covered?

Medicare (Original)
Part A (covered inpatient care in hospitals)
Part B (covered outpatient care and medical services)

Private health insurance
Medicare pays for covered benefits first   (Primary)
Insurance may pay some of the remainder   (Secondary)

What aspects of Medicare are not covered?

Medicare Part C
(Medicare Advantage Plans managed by private insurance companies)

Medicare Part D
(Drug Benefit)

Medigap Insurance
(Private or public Medicare supplemental policies)

For all Medicare plans, see Medicare And You, 2010

http://www.medicare.gov/Publications/Pubs/pdf/10050.pdf

My loved one has Medicare, so is he eligible for every benefit?

A Medicare recipient is not automatically entitled to every benefit. Your loved one may be covered for home healthcare durable medical equipment (DME) (page 74) like a home healthcare bed, wheelchair and walker, but may not qualify for the Medicare Home Health Benefit (page 58) for visiting nurses and therapists. Coverage depends on your loved one qualifying under the provision a benefit is offered.

<u>Medicare Or Insurance, Who Pays First?</u>

Who pays a claim first, Medicare or insurance?

Many insurance company plans follow Medicare as secondary, but ask your company to be sure. You can also refer to a Medicare information booklet, Who Pays First. It explains how Medicare works with other kinds of insurance or coverage.

http://www.medicare.gov/Publications/Pubs/pdf/02179.pdf

What is primary and secondary insurance?

A secondary insurer considers the remainder of a claim after the primary pays all or part of the claim or denies coverage. A secondary may pay a large part of the remaining portion of a covered claim after the primary insurer (typically, Medicare) pays its share.

A secondary may not pay anything if the primary insurer does not cover the claim as part of the benefit plan or if the primary denies payment for something usually covered.

So a secondary never pays if the primary doesn't cover the claim?

It depends on the insurer and what they choose to cover. Medicare never covers at home intravenous (IV) antibiotics, so a private plan may not pay either. But for some goods and services, if Medicare denies coverage, insurance may pay a portion. If your insurance plan is a secondary and Medicare denies payment for a "never covered" good or service, ask your insurance if they will cover some of it anyway.

Medicare Providers

What is a provider?

A provider is an entity providing medical care, medical services, medical equipment or medical supplies. They either collect payment at the time of delivery/service or submit claims to Medicare and insurance and bill your loved one later for anything owed and unpaid.

Why should I care about providers? What should I be careful about?

The amount ultimately owed depends on the relationship the provider has with Medicare, so ask each provider if they are enrolled and participate in Medicare.

What are important Medicare terms and how do they relate to how much my loved one has to pay?

It's worth your time to understand these basic concepts to save the most money, find mistakes in your loved one's favor and not be taken advantage of.

Enrolled, participating and accepting assignment
The provider has signed an agreement to "accept" Medicare payments for covered goods and services up to Medicare allowed amounts, so they can bill your loved one only for the difference, if any, between the allowed amount and what Medicare paid toward it. Providers are not allowed to bill for the entire difference between what Medicare paid them and their (higher) uninsured rate. If Medicare denies coverage, your loved one is liable to the provider for no more than the allowed amount.

Paying at the time of service
A provider, in most cases, cannot collect more than 20% of the allowed amount for a covered good or service. The standard Medicare reimbursement is 80% of the allowed amount, so if your loved one is required to pay 20% to the provider at the time of service, it is usually the balance to be owed anyway. The provider submits to Medicare for the remaining 80% of the allowed amount.

If insurance follows Medicare as a secondary
If possible, use providers who don't require any payment at the time of delivery and will submit a claim to insurance as well as Medicare, which pays 80% of the allowed amount, so insurance can have a chance to pay part of the 20%.

I like this provider, so my loved one will agree to pay 20% at the time of service.

In that case, save the receipts and compare them to the quarterly Medicare statement (MSN) to verify your loved one didn't pay the provider more than 20% of the allowed amount. If he did, then after Medicare has paid 80% of the allowed amount, get a refund from the provider for the difference between 20% of the allowed amount and what your loved one paid at the time of service.

Can a provider ever collect 100% at delivery?

If it is "made to order" or costs less than $150
In this case, the provider is permitted to require your loved
one to pay 100% of the Medicare allowed amount upon
delivery of the covered equipment, but if they do, they must
submit a claim to Medicare on your loved one's behalf (page
80) for 80% of the allowed amount.

If Medicare NEVER covers the good or service
With no expectation of coverage, a provider may collect up to
100% of the allowed amount at delivery and doesn't have to
submit a claim (page 81).

Does the provider charge a delivery fee?

Medicare doesn't cover delivery fees. Some providers charge
for delivery, so it's wise to ask.

The Advance Beneficiary Notice

What am I signing at the time of service?

A provider who intends to bill Medicare and/or insurance
may, as a condition of providing the good or service,
require at the time of delivery, the signature of an Advance
Beneficiary Notice (ABN), also called:

"Assignment Of Benefits And Waiver Of Liability"

A provider will require a signature if Medicare usually covers
the good or service, but in your loved one's situation, there
is uncertainly Medicare will pay the claim. If Medicare never

covers the good or service or if it is paid in full at delivery, they don't need a signed ABN.

A signature allows the provider to submit your loved one's private information to Medicare and insurance. You are on notice your loved one has to pay whatever Medicare and/or insurance don't cover up to their allowed amounts and if a provider needs additional information for submission, like a certification of medical necessity from the doctor, it is your responsibility to get it to the provider.

The Sequence Of A Claim Submission

With Medicare as the primary, what is the sequence of a provider submitting a claim?

The provider submits a claim to Medicare
Medicare processes the claim and pays its share of the allowed amount or denies it. It usually takes six weeks, but can take longer. If it is denied, follow up with the provider to find out why and ask if supplying additional documentation, like a certification of medical necessity, will reopen the claim or if you will need to file an appeal (pages 212-213).

Medicare sends an MSN
Every three months, Medicare generates a statement called a Medicare Summary Notice (MSN) and mails a copy to your loved one (the beneficiary or insured person) and to the submitting provider. Check the statement to verify the providers who delivered covered goods and/or services have submitted claims. A claim may not show up until you receive the next MSN, but in the meantime, you can call the provider to find out when it was submitted and its status.

The provider also submits to insurance
While Medicare processes the claim, the provider also submits a claim to insurance, but insurance acting as a secondary won't complete processing it until they know how much Medicare will or won't pay and why. After Medicare pays 80% of the allowed amount, insurance may pay up to 80% of the remaining 20%.

Insurance sends an EOB
After insurance receives the claim submission, they generate a statement called an Explanation Of Benefits (EOB) and send copies to your loved one and the provider. The EOB may show the claim as fully processed or indicate a request for additional information from the provider such as a copy of the Medicare statement (MSN) pertaining to the claim, a request for a certification of medical necessity (issued by the doctor) or it may state the claim was denied and list the reasons for denial.

Insurance waits for the Medicare statement
In most cases, the provider must send a copy of the Medicare Summary Notice (MSN) to insurance acting as a secondary. Until insurance receives the MSN showing Medicare fully processed the claim, they will put a pending status on the submitted file.

If too much time passes waiting for the MSN, insurance may send your loved one an EOB denying its share of the claim, making your loved one potentially responsible to the provider for any remaining balance up to the Medicare allowed amount. Call the provider and ask them to send a copy of the MSN to insurance. It's routine for a copy of an MSN to take a while to get from a provider to insurance, so the denial of a claim for lack of a requested MSN does not necessarily mean insurance won't eventually pay when they finally get the MSN.

Insurance sends an updated EOB statement
An updated Explanation Of Benefits (EOB) may show the claim as still in process, a request for additional information, a notification of payments to the provider or indicate a denial. If Medicare and insurance have paid their shares, the EOB will show the reminder of the Medicare allowed amount for which the provider can bill your loved one.

Your loved one receives a bill from the provider
After Medicare and insurance have paid their shares toward the claim, the bill received from the provider should match the remaining amount due on the EOB, which may say, "(Provider Name) May Bill You: $" (the remainder of the allowed amount, if any).

You may need to follow up
If your copy of the Medicare Summary Notice (MSN) doesn't show a good or service submitted to Medicare at all, call the provider to find out if and when the provider submitted it.

If the MSN shows the claim in process, but the insurance Explanation Of Benefits (EOB) statement has a footnote saying the insurance company needs "additional information", ask insurance if their EOB is referring to a copy of an MSN they have not yet received or to some other documentation, like a certification of medical necessity from the doctor.

For more help with the Medicare Summary Notice (MSN) Part A and Part B:

http://www.medicare.gov/Basics/SummaryNotice_HowToRead.asp

<u>Following Up On Provider Claim Submissions</u>

How do I know providers are submitting claims to insurance as well as Medicare?

Your loved one may receive a bill from a provider after Medicare has processed the claim, but the remaining balance may not have been submitted to or fully processed by insurance.

Billing your loved one before a claim is fully processed is usually by mistake, but some providers may skip billing Medicare and/or insurance and send your loved one the bill, hoping to receive a direct payment.

If a provider bills your loved one and you have an MSN showing completion of Medicare processing, but don't have an EOB, ask the provider for evidence of claim processing by insurance. They can send you a copy of the EOB. If they don't have it, tell them your loved one will not pay until you have an EOB showing the claim as fully processed with a final balance.

What can I do to confirm a provider has submitted a claim to Medicare?

If you receive a provider bill for a Medicare covered good or service without evidence of submission for reimbursement and don't see claim submission data on the current quarterly MSN, call the provider and ask them when they submitted the claim. If the submission information for the claim is not on the next Medicare statement three months later, call the provider again. If you are not satisfied, tell them you may call 800 MEDICARE to make a complaint that you are being billed by a provider who is not first submitting to Medicare.

Do I need to make sure providers submit their Medicare claims?

If they bill your loved one for covered goods and services without submitting to Medicare first, tell them to submit to Medicare. If the Medicare statements you receive have entries showing Medicare submission, the process is moving forward and you don't owe a specific amount yet.

But, follow up on claims for covered durable medical equipment (DME) your loved one had to pay for in full at delivery (because the cost was under $150 or the equipment was made to order) to make sure they are submitted to Medicare on your loved one's behalf (page 80).

What about late provider claims for Medicare covered goods or services?

As long as you are not being billed yet, I wouldn't bother a provider to submit a Medicare claim for his own reimbursement. If a provider fails to submit a Medicare claim within one year of the date of service, the maximum they can bill Medicare (or your loved one, if Medicare denies the claim) is 10% of the Medicare allowed amount.

If the provider submits within the one year limit, the most he can bill your loved one, assuming Medicare pays 80% of the allowed amount, is 20%.

Where can I go for more answers about Medicare?

See the following sites (and Appendix 7):

Medicare
(U.S. Department of Health and Human Services)

http://www.medicare.gov

Medicare And You, 2010
(U.S. Department of Health and Human Services)

http://www.medicare.gov/Publications/Pubs/pdf/10050.pdf

The Medicare Interactive Topic Menu
(Medicare Rights Center)

http://www.medicareinteractive.com/page2.php?topic=counselor&page
=Index#III

Issues With Provider Bills Sent To Your Loved One

At what point should I pay a bill for covered goods and services from a provider?

The most important steps are receiving copies of Medicare and insurance statements (MSN and EOB) for the claim and examining them to be sure they agree with the provider's billed amount.

Don't pay anything if you are still waiting for the MSN and EOB or if they don't agree with the amount billed to your loved one. Call the provider to let them know you want to help the process of getting coverage determined and your loved one will pay the balance due after complete processing by Medicare and insurance.

If the statements show the claim as fully processed and the amount remaining due from your loved one as stated on the

EOB is equal to the amount on the bill, it needs to be paid.

The Amount Due notice from a provider seems like a bill and a statement in one. What should I do?

A statement is sent to display the status of your loved one's medical expenses and submitted claims and as notification your loved one might owe some or all of the expenses, once coverage has been decided. A bill is sent to collect a final amount due after a claim has been fully processed by Medicare and/or insurance.

When a provider sends your loved one a statement for Medicare or insurance covered goods and services, it may have graphics and language to cause it to be mistaken for a bill. Your copies of the MSN and the EOB are clear about medical expenses submitted as claims and what your loved one owes the provider, so always refer to them.

Does it matter if the provider regards the document I received as a statement or a bill?

If the provider considers it a bill, they expect to be paid soon. If they consider it a statement, the claim is still in process, so no payment from your loved one is due yet. To the extent you want to stay on the right side of the provider, it is helpful to know what the provider expects from the document they sent. Call the provider and ask them.

What about intimidating or confusing billing language appearing on the same document?

Don't pay until you refer to the MSN and EOB to see if the stated amount owed by your loved one agrees with the provider's bill. Call the provider to find out the intent of the bill or statement and explain your loved one won't pay until you have an MSN and EOB. If they have an MSN and EOB relating to the expenses, ask them to send copies to you.

Don't be confused or intimidated by ambiguous or harsh billing language, usually in large or bold type, including the following "billing-ese":

"HOSPITAL BILL" in large, faint lettering overlaying an itemized list of medical expenses and claim processing activity.

"Your account shows a balance of $. Please remit payment by (date)."

"Your account is past due in the amount of $. Please remit payment by (date)." (30 days later)

"Final Notice! To avoid collection action, which may include agency assignment, remit balance due immediately." (Another 30 days later)

Instead, look for fine print on the same statement, which indicates claim processing is not complete and your loved one is not yet expected to pay, for example:

"This is not a bill. Your insurance is being billed."

"Please note Your Responsibility is estimated and is subject to change based upon your insurance carrier's final claim determination."

Medicare has processed the claim, but insurance hasn't sent me an EOB showing the submission. I have received a bill from the provider, which says they have billed insurance. How can this be?

Watch for fine print like this on provider bills:

"We have billed all known insurance and this amount is now due."

"All known insurance" doesn't necessarily mean private insurance as well as Medicare was billed. It can mean only Medicare was billed.

Make sure both Medicare and insurance have been billed and both have fully processed the claim. The only way to know this is to receive the MSN and EOB and check the amount due against the provider's bill.

I keep getting Past Due notices from a provider.

Some providers may try to rush payment by stamping "Past Due" or "Seriously Past Due" on every outgoing bill or statement, even if the payment is not late. If you get a Past Due stamped notice arriving before the MSN and EOB, call the provider to ask why they consider it past due.

The provider tells me it is a bill and is due because the claim was denied.

If a claim was denied, ask why. Do they need additional information from your loved one or from the doctor to resubmit? Tell the provider you are not going to pay until you have MSN and EOB statements showing the claim was submitted with all required and requested information proving the processing is complete. In the meantime, discuss what you can do to help, so Medicare and insurance can fully process the claim.

A provider says Medicare is denying the claim and my most recent Medicare statement shows this. What can I do?

Don't panic and don't pay the provider yet.

Is the claim for something Medicare NEVER covers?
There is no benefit to making an appeal to Medicare, but make sure the provider submits the claim to insurance with copies of the MSN showing the denial. In some instances, insurance will make a payment toward the denied Medicare claim. After insurance decides and you have the MSN and the EOB, your loved one owes whatever was not paid up to the allowed amount.

Is the claim for something Medicare SOMETIMES covers?
Call the provider's billing office to say you want to do whatever you can to get Medicare (and insurance) to cover it, but after you exhaust all avenues, your loved one will pay the balance due up to the allowed amount. You may need to ask the doctor for a certification of medical necessity.

The provider can appeal a decision.
If Medicare denies all or a portion of a claim, the provider may appeal the decision. After the appeal is decided, the provider may bill your loved one for the balance up to the allowed amount.

You can appeal a Medicare claim denial.
The deadline to appeal a Medicare decision is within 120 days of receipt of the MSN showing the denial. For more information, see:

Medicare And You, 2010: How To File An Appeal.
(web pdf pages 86-88)

http://www.medicare.gov/Publications/Pubs/pdf/10050.pdf

U.S. Department of Health and Human Services
(Medicare Appeals and Grievances)

http://www.medicare.gov/basics/appeals.asp

Why would Medicare reverse a denial of coverage?

If a medical condition worsens, it can create a medical
necessity for additional complex and expensive goods and
services. These extras may be denied if Medicare is not
yet aware of the change in medical condition since the last
similar claim. If Medicare makes payment, but excludes the
extras, appeal the decision and provide documentation.

Additional Common Billing Issues

What are some typical problems with bills?

Multiple bills for the same claim
Most providers generate bills automatically, so if payments
and bills cross in the mail, your loved one may receive bills
already paid. Call the provider's billing office to be sure the
bill was actually paid.

A payment isn't credited to the account
If a provider doesn't credit a payment to your loved one's
account, don't ignore the bills and wait for them to discover
and correct the oversight. Call them to clear it up.

Bills your loved one shouldn't receive
Maybe your loved one shouldn't have been billed at all, because Medicare and/or insurance already paid all of it. Or, maybe the provider's contract with Medicare or insurance doesn't allow them to bill for that expense (page 216).

Bills arriving too soon
Soon after your loved one comes home from the hospital, you may receive a long hospital bill. Don't let it scare you. It may be far too soon to have been submitted to and fully processed by both Medicare and insurance. If you have not received an MSN or EOB, your loved one doesn't owe anything yet.

Over-billing for late Medicare submissions
There is a Medicare deadline that works in your loved one's favor. The provider must bill Medicare within one year of the date of service or the maximum amount due from Medicare (or your loved one if the claim is denied) is 10% of the allowed amount. If Medicare covers the late claim and pays the provider 10% of the allowed amount, the provider must accept it as final. If Medicare denies payment, your loved one owes the provider only 10% of the allowed amount. If the 10% is worth the effort, find out why Medicare denied it and see if you can reverse the denial, so Medicare will pay the 10%. Otherwise, pay the provider the 10%.

Late insurance claim submissions
Private insurance companies have provider deadlines for submission of claims, for completing a claim submission and supplying requested additional information. Some insurance companies have 90-day, six month and one-year limits for submission by contracted providers, such as hospitals. If a claim is submitted after the deadline and the delay is not excused due to an acceptable reason, insurance may deny the claim and the provider may have to absorb the bill.

The provider says insurance is not responding
If you get a provider statement showing an old claim, call the provider's billing office and ask how you can help. If they say insurance has not responded, but you have no EOBs after all this time, call insurance and have them look into it. It could be they have no record of the submission, because the claim was submitted with a wrong ID number.

You didn't read the EOB
When you receive an EOB, read it carefully, so you will not miss a request from insurance for additional information. If you see this, call the provider and make sure they have everything they need to complete the claim submission.

If insurance makes a request for additional information on a submitted claim and too much time passes from the time you receive the EOB showing the request, they may deny the claim and your loved one may become responsible for payment. If a claim is denied because of the delay, insurance may re-open it after receiving the requested information or may require an appeal.

I'm getting hospital bills from more than one source. What should I watch for?

Duplicate billings on outsourced statements
Monthly hospital statements may contain billing entries from some of your loved one's doctors and other providers. Other hospital based providers and some doctors attending your loved one's case may instead use private billing companies to submit claims and mail their bills. An outsourced bill can have duplicate charges of a hospital bill, so check by comparing bill entries from these different billing sources by date of service. You may find entries on an outsourced bill you have already been billed for by the hospital.

Denied charges outsourced and billed

You may receive bills that show amounts due, but are not really owed, because as stated on the EOB, the charges are "not a billable expense and not owed" by your loved one per the insurance company contract with the hospital. Some hospitals outsource part of their bill processing and billing, so it's possible the hospital may send a claim for disallowed charges to an outside billing company to bill your loved one. If you don't pay attention to each EOB and match them with your bills, you might overpay. Call insurance and ask them to call the hospital to straighten it out.

I called the private billing company about a charge from one of our doctors, but I can't get them to help me.

Tell the billing company you want to discuss the bill, but your loved one will not pay anything unless they speak with you. Tell them you will call the doctor, their client, to say his billing company is not being responsive to requests from the family about a bill. If you have to, call the doctor's office and have them call the billing company to request they speak with you.

The illness is long over, but months later there are statements and bills still coming from providers. How can I be sure I'm nearing the end of it?

After the illness is over, providers are no longer delivering goods and services, but statements and bills from submitted and processed Medicare and insurance claims can trickle in for many months. Call each provider and request a statement that includes every remaining date of service, so you can be aware of all the remaining possible claims and bills coming from each provider.

What is a super statement?

This is a summary statement from a provider showing all goods and services delivered to your loved one, submitted claims and payments from Medicare and insurance to the provider and payments from your loved one from the first claim at the beginning of the illness to the present.

Providers don't like sending super statements, because they don't want to make it easy for you to examine the billing history where you might find mistakes, duplicate billings or ask complex time-consuming questions about differences in charges, reimbursements and why billed amounts varied with similar claims.

If you have been receiving confusing bills over a long period, request a super statement and the opportunity to go over it with them. Sometimes, the request will make the billing office take you seriously and address your concerns. If they won't send one, get all your statement copies together and tell the provider you want to meet with them before paying anything more.

How can I keep track of bills and payments?

If you write the statement number on your loved one's payment check and staple a copy of the check to a copy of the bill and clip it to the MSN and EOB showing the corresponding claim, months later you will be able to find them easily.

A daily journal (page 119) comes in handy to recall events surrounding the date of service and is a great way to track events and conversations as well as the dates surrounding received goods and services. Using a simple bookkeeping program like Quicken makes it easy to record and track expenses.

<u>Dealing With An Insurance Company</u>

How can I deal with the insurance company, so I don't get the run-around?

If you can't get a competent person on the phone or you get a new person every time you call, start at the top and work down. If your loved one has a group plan sponsored by an employer, ask the group administrator to call the insurance company and speak to the person in charge of customer service about getting things moving.

Can I get one person assigned to my case?

Ask the customer service manager to assign a customer service agent or a nurse case manager to oversee your loved one's case. From then on, when you call your assigned person's direct line, you will be speaking with someone familiar with your loved one's medical and claim history.

The insurance statement (EOB) shows a claim as "pending". It says they require "additional information" or it says, "Your claim was denied because the requested information was not received". What do these comments mean?

Insurance (acting as a secondary) could be waiting for a copy of the Medicare statement (MSN) from the provider, because before they finish processing, they want to know if Medicare has paid or denied the claim. Insurance gives the provider plenty of time to send a copy of an MSN, but don't assume "additional information" on the EOB always refers to Medicare statements. Insurance might need a certification of medical necessity. Call insurance to find out, because it is up to your loved one to get the appropriate documents to the provider and to insurance.

My insurance company says they have all they need to process the claim, but it's been months.

The insurer could be delaying payment on a fully processed claim to collect interest on the money they owe your loved one. Some states have prompt payment laws to penalize a private insurer if the insurer doesn't pay the claim within a certain period of time. Some of these states have sought to strengthen their laws by tightening the definitions of a "clean claim", barring plans from overriding prompt-pay time limits, and by trying to define exactly when a claim is deemed as being paid. Consider calling the insurance commissioner's office of your state to get the latest regulations and laws for this matter. For a state by state listing of prompt payment laws and regulations:

http://www.justmypassion.com/files/Prompt_Pay_State_Grid.pdf

Phone Conversation Tips

Why are you giving me tips about using the phone?

When dealing with receptionists, office assistants, nurses, doctors, hospital billing, laboratories, home healthcare departments, insurance companies, home healthcare supply companies and others, half the battle is effective communication. With better communication, you will expend less effort, suffer less stress, receive better care, save time and sometimes, money.

The person tells me they will "handle it", but when I call back, I get a different person who has no record of my request.

It sounds basic, but remember to get the first and last name of the person with whom you are speaking and write it down along with what you requested and what the person said. If you don't, the next person will probably ask you, "Who did you speak to?" and you will have to start over. Every time you call to make an appointment, to get an estimated time of arrival (ETA) and when you confirm or request anything, get the name of the person giving you information. Even when the person confirms or verifies information to your satisfaction, get the name in case the person has made a mistake.

If you don't have the name of the person, he will feel less accountable for mistakes or not following up. Errors from carelessness are fewer when a person on the other end of the line knows you have his name.

The person on the other end doesn't give a name.

A conversation should not begin until you have the person's name or ID number and phone extension or direct number. If the person won't or isn't allowed to give you the extension, direct number or last name, ask if she is the only Mary or if he is the only Joe at that number, so you don't get the "Which Mary?" or the "We have three Joe's here..." routine when you call back. Ask if there is a unique ID number the person can give you for reference.

When I call back, the person I need "just left for the day".

During your first call, ask the person helping you if he will still be on duty and available during the entire time the issue is supposed to be resolved. For same-day resolutions, ask until what time he is working. He might, after having just told you he will take care of it and call you before he leaves say, "Oh yeah, I am leaving before lunch today and won't be returning until Monday". If follow up is expected to occur over the next couple of days or during the following week, ask what days he regularly works, if that is his upcoming schedule and, if not, who fills in for him.

I get handed off to another person and have to start over.

If the person helping you will not be working until the close of business, find out who will be assigned his tasks. Don't rely on the first person putting your request "in the notes" on the computer to let the next person know about it. The relief person might not see the notes or do your request last. Speak with the relief person as well and make sure he understands the time frame you have been promised. Be nice if you want him to make an effort.

What about businesses with multiple call centers?

Some 800 numbers go to different geographical locations due to time of day and/or call load, so ask if the number dials into only one call center location. If not, ask the person helping you how he refers to his call center, so later you can say you spoke with so and so at such and such location to reach him or someone filling in for him.

I call a provider to clarify a situation, but keep getting put on hold.

Leave a polite message with the provider saying there is no way your loved one will pay until you are able to speak with someone and resolve the issue. They will become available to discuss your concerns.

What if I call, but they are closed?

The first time you do business with them, get the hours of operation and put them in your Home Healthcare Contact Information List (Appendix 2). Ask the person if the same number will get him throughout the entire shift or if you need to call an after hours number. Whenever you get an answering service, say, "I need the back line". Sometimes, this will get your call directed to a person who can help you.

Acknowledgements

My family and I would like to express our gratitude to UCLA Medical Center and the attending physicians for their patience, kindness and professionalism with special mention:

Jon Kobashigawa MD and fellow cardiologists:

Jaime Moriguchi MD, Michele Hamilton MD, Antoine Hage MD, Jignesh Patel MD PhD, Michelle Kittleson MD

Hillel Laks MD, Cardiothoracic Surgery

Michael Levine MD, Pulmonology

Ardis Moe MD, Infectious Disease

Marvin Bergsneider MD, Neurosurgery

My family and I also thank the nurses and caregivers who provided bedside care and shared their love with Mom.

Thank you to those who encouraged me to develop this handbook and for their time and advice:

Martin Levin Esq., literary attorney
Digby Diehl, author and literary critic
Rich Barber, literary agent
Jerry Gross, book editor, Independent Editors Group
Eric Marton, President/CEO California Heart Center
Christine Sumbi, Vice-President California Heart Center

In Appreciation Of Nurses

Nurses have a very, very tough job.

Nurses are the "primary healers" and make the difference in your loved one's chances, especially with acute cases.

Nurses work long hours and are on their feet most of the time. They work past the point of exhaustion.

They must respond to urgencies and emergencies and still take care of their routine tasks.

They are between the doctor and the family. They must remain calm when family members lose their composure.

They translate care from the physician to the patient by effecting doctor's orders, while using judgment and experience to make adjustments to changing conditions.

Nurses are trained to be patient advocates, so learn from them and form a relationship based on advocacy. Appreciate their efforts by giving them the respect they deserve.

I will always be grateful for their kindness and professionalism.

James Thomas Williams

Appendix 1

Hospital Information List

Doctor Information List

Primary care physician name and specialty
Colleagues' names and schedule rotation
Other attending physicians
When each doctor is usually on duty and on call
Times they usually do daily rounds
When each is to be away on vacation
Office addresses, phone, fax, pager numbers, email addresses

Nurse Information List

Hospital unit manager name and phone number
Nurse supervisor name and phone number
Charge nurse name and phone number
Nurse's station phone number
Nurses attending your loved one

Emergency Room (ER)

Street directions to ER
Visitor parking and walking directions to ER
ER phone number
ER doctors and nurses attending your loved one

Hospital Admissions

Location of Admissions Office in the hospital
Admissions person name and phone number

Unit, floor and room

Unit name (e.g. CCU, ICU, Recovery), floor number and wing
Room number and directions to the room
Room phone number
Visiting hours

Dieticians

Supervising dietician name
Your loved one's dietician name
Office phone, fax, pager numbers, email addresses

Hospital parking

Street directions to main hospital parking lot or structure
Walking directions from the parking lot to the hospital room
Cost per day and multi-day or monthly permit discounts
Where to purchase discount parking permits
Free, lower cost or street parking alternatives

Discharge

Discharge coordinator name
Office phone, fax and pager numbers, email address
Cell phone number

Hospital Laboratory

Hours and directions to laboratory drop-off desk
Directions to main hospital lab (if drop-off desk is closed)
Short term free parking for drop-offs
(After your loved one comes home, you may have to take
samples to the laboratory for analysis)

Appendix 2

Home Healthcare Contact Information List

Neighbors

Names, addresses, phone numbers and email addresses
Order of priority (ask them first) to contact in the event of an emergency, after you call 911

Private ambulance company (not 911)

(Medicare and insurance may cover non-emergency medical transport from home to the hospital and back for a medically necessary reason)

Company name, main phone and fax number and the after hours phone number
Manager and dispatcher names and phone extensions
Make sure they cover your area

Home healthcare companies

Customer service and technical support numbers and the after hours numbers
Dispatcher name and direct line number and the after hours phone number
Names and cell numbers of technicians who visit the residence and what they deliver and set up (e.g. oxygen equipment, disposable supplies)
Equipment and supplies provided by each company

Internet vendors

Website addresses, products purchased and frequency
Owner and manager names and email addresses
800 numbers, time zones
Shipping deadlines, terms and discounts

Specialty pharmacies and retail drug stores

Pharmacy street address
Managing pharmacist's name
Main phone number, pharmacy phone, fax and after hours
pharmacy number
Days of the week and hours of operation and days/hours for
pharmacy deliveries (they might be different)
Daily deadlines for same day prescription deliveries
Delivery charges, if any
Prescription and non-prescription products provided by each
pharmacy

Mobile X-ray company

Main phone and fax number
Manager and dispatcher names
After hours company phone number
Visiting technician name and cell number
Radiologist after hours phone number
Make sure they cover your area

Visiting nurses and therapists

Agency or hospital department name
Owner or manager and assistant name
Main phone and after hours numbers
Names and cell numbers of nurses who regularly visit

Visiting nurses' visit schedules

Names and cell phone numbers:

Physical Therapists   (PT)
Occupational Therapists   (OT)
Speech Therapists   (ST)

Therapists' visit schedules

Insurance

Insurance company name, mailing address and 800 number
Claims processing center mailing address and 800 number
Group and membership number
Policy type (HMO, PPO, POS)
Group name (company providing the insurance)

Group administrator name
Customer service manager
Direct lines (or extensions), fax and cell numbers and email
addresses

Other home healthcare contacts

Name and title of contacts
Company names and mailing addresses
Hospital affiliations, if any
Phone, pager, cell phone, fax numbers and email addresses

Appendix 3

Medicine Chart

MEDICATION RECORD

1 Time	2 Initial	3 Site Inj. Comment	1 Time	2 Initial	3 Site Inj. Comment
4 PRN Med. Reason/Response			4 PRN Med. Reason/Response		

CODE FOR SITE OF INJECTION	GLUTEAL	LATEROFEMORAL	ABDOMEN-LOWER
	LG-Left	LF-Left	AB-RUQ-Right upper quadrant
	RG-Right	RF-Right	AB-LUQ-Left upper quadrant
	VENTROGLUTEAL	DELTOID	AB-RLQ-Right lower quadrant
	LV-Left	LA-Left	AB-LLQ-Left lower quadrant
	RV-Right	RA-Right	

ALLERGIES:

RN/ RTE	MEDICATION – DOSE – SCHEDULE	START/STOP	ADMINISTERED DOSES

SIGNATURE = initials as above plus signature

Appendix 4

Excerpts From Music/Stroke Study

Regarding stroke patients, a study at Helsinki University between March 2004 and May 2006 reports that music alone has shown to have a significant positive effect on victims of brain injury such as stroke. The study showed that 3 months after a cerebral artery stroke, music listeners had double the improvement in verbal memory than did non-listeners. The differences in results held true for 6 months. The listeners also experienced less depression than non-listeners.

"As a result of our findings, we suggest that everyday music listening during early stroke recovery offers a valuable addition to the patients' care-especially if other active forms of rehabilitation are not yet feasible at this stage-by providing an individually targeted, easy-to-conduct and inexpensive means to facilitate cognitive and emotional recovery," says Teppo Särkämö, the first author of the study.

"Other research has shown that during the first weeks and months after stroke, the patients typically spend about three-quarters of their time each day in non-therapeutic activities, mostly in their rooms, inactive and without interaction, even although this time-window is ideal for rehabilitative training from the point of view of brain plasticity. Our research shows for the first time that listening to music during this crucial period can enhance cognitive recovery and prevent negative mood, and it has the advantage that it is cheap and easy to organize," Särkämö concludes.

Oxford University Press Journal, February 2008

Appendix 5

Y Port Tube Feeding Adapter Ordering

Boston Scientific   Customer Service: 888 272-1001
Endo Vive
Y-Port Feeding Adapter
REF/Catalogue No. 8064
U.P.N. M00580640 20 Fr.

"For use with initial and replacement gastronomy tube".

Boston Scientific does not sell directly to patients.
One of their distributors, Applied Medical, takes MasterCard
and Visa, but does not bill Medicare or insurance.

Applied Medical   Customer service: 800 869-7382
8000 Katherine Boulevard
Brecksville, Ohio 44141

Part number: 4-2020

http://www.appliedmedical.net/

Apria Healthcare is a nationwide home healthcare company.
They can order from Applied Medical and bill Medicare and
insurance:

Apria Healthcare   Customer service: 800 277-4288
26220 Enterprise Court
Lake Forest, CA 92630

http://www.apria.com/branch_locator1/1,3577,496-California,00.html

Appendix 6

U.S. Government
Health Information Websites

**U.S. Department of Health and Human Services
Administration on Aging**

"The mission of the Administration on Aging (AoA) is to help elderly individuals maintain their dignity and independence in their homes and communities through comprehensive, coordinated, and cost effective systems of long-term care, and livable communities across the U.S."

http://www.aoa.gov/

Medicines And You: A Guide For Older Adults

Council on Family Health "in cooperation with U.S. Department of Health and Human Services Food and Drug Administration and the Administration on Aging"

http://www.aging.state.pa.us/aging/lib/aging/Medicines_and_You.pdf

U.S. Department of Health and Human Services

"The Department of Health and Human Services (HHS) is the United States government's principal agency for protecting the health of all Americans and providing essential human services, especially for those who are least able to help themselves."

http://www.hhs.gov/

U.S. Department of Health and Human Services
Nursing Home Compare

"Find And Compare Nursing Homes"

http://www.medicare.gov/NHCompare/Include/DataSection/
Questions/SearchCriteriaNEW.asp?version=default&browser=IE%7C7%
7CWinXP&language=English&defaultstatus=0&pagelist=Home&Cookies
EnabledStatus=True

U.S. Food and Drug Administration
Department of Health and Human Services

"The FDA is responsible for protecting the public health
by assuring the safety, efficacy, and security of human and
veterinary drugs, biological products, medical devices, our
nation's food supply, cosmetics, and products that emit
radiation."

http://www.fda.gov/

Appendix 7

Medicare Information Websites

Medicare

U.S. Department of Health and Human Services

http://www.medicare.gov/

Medicare And You, 2010

"The official government handbook with important information about the following: What's new, 2010 Medicare costs, What Medicare covers, Health and prescription drug plans, Your Medicare rights, Fraud and identity theft."

http://www.medicare.gov/Publications/Pubs/pdf/10050.pdf

Medicare and Other Health Benefits: Your Guide to Who Pays First

"This official government booklet tells you: How Medicare works with other types of insurance or coverage, Who should pay your bills first, Where to get more help."

http://www.medicare.gov/Publications/Pubs/pdf/02179.pdf

Medicare Rights Center

"The Medicare Rights Center is a national, nonprofit consumer service organization that works to ensure access to affordable health care for older adults and people with disabilities through counseling and advocacy, educational programs and public policy initiatives. Since 1989, we've been helping people with Medicare understand their rights and benefits, navigate the Medicare system and secure the quality care they deserve."

http://www.medicarerights.org/

Medicare Interactive

"A free, independent online resource brought to you by the Medicare Rights Center, puts a world of clear, timely guidance about Medicare benefits and options right at your fingertips"

http://www.medicareinteractive.org/index.php

The Medicare Interactive Topic Menu

http://www.medicareinteractive.com/page2.php?topic=counselor&page=Index#III

What does Medicare Part A Cover?

http://www.medicareinteractive.org/page2.php?topic=counselor&page=script&slide_id=178

What does Medicare Part B Cover?
(Includes Durable Medical Equipment)

http://www.medicareinteractive.org/page2.php?topic=counselor&page=script&slide_id=170

What is not covered by Medicare?

http://www.medicareinteractive.org/page2.php?topic=counselor&page=script&slide_id=215

What is Durable Medical Equipment DME?

http://www.medicareinteractive.org/page2.php?topic=counselor&page=script&slide_id=188

What does not qualify as durable medical equipment (DME)?

http://www.medicareinteractive.org/page2.php?topic=counselor&page=script&slide_id=1570

How to read your Medicare Summary Notice (MSN) Part A (sample Part A MSN):

http://www.medicare.gov/Basics/SummaryNotice_HowToRead.asp

How to read your Medicare Summary Notice (MSN) Part B (sample Part B MSN):

http://www.medicare.gov/Basics/SummaryNotice_HowToReadB.asp

Medicare Appeals and Grievances:

http://www.medicare.gov/basics/appeals.asp

View and download Medicare appeals forms:

http://www.medicare.gov/basics/forms/default.asp

Appendix 8

NLM And NIH Websites

The following websites and information are a service of the U.S. National Library of Medicine (NLM) and the National Institutes of Health (NIH). To learn more about clinical trials and the state of professional and researcher knowledge, consult these sites and those in Appendix 9.

MEDLINE Plus

A user friendly site for the public dedicated to health isssues:

http://medlineplus.gov/

MEDLINE Plus has links to search databases of clinical trials:

http://clinicaltrials.gov/

MEDLINE Plus also has links to other NLM and NIH databases, Federal Government resources and other health organization databases:

http://www.nlm.nih.gov/medlineplus/databases.html

PubMed

Over 18 million citations from MEDLINE and other life science journals for biomedical articles back to 1948.

The result of a MEDLINE/PubMed search is a list of citations (including authors, title, source, and often an abstract) to journal articles and an indication of free electronic full-text availability:

http://www.pubmed.gov

or

http://www.ncbi.nlm.nih.gov/pubmed/

NLM Gateway

MEDLINE in PubMed may also be searched using the "NLM Gateway", a single Web interface that searches multiple NLM retrieval systems to allow users to initiate searches from one Web interface, providing "one-stop searching" for many of NLM's information resources or databases:

http://gateway.nlm.nih.gov/gw/Cmd

Appendix 9

Additional Research/Healthcare Websites

To learn about clinical trials and the state of professional and researcher knowledge, see sites listed here and Appendix 8.

Research!America

"A not for profit membership supported alliance advocating biomedical research performed by public and private institutions on behalf of donor organizations including the Federal government with special emphasis on the National Institutes of Health, Bethesda Maryland."

http://www.researchamerica.org/

The National Institutes of Health (NIH)

"Part of the U.S. Department of Health and Human Services, NIH is the primary Federal agency for conducting and supporting medical research. NIH is the steward of medical and behavioral research for the Nation. Its mission is science in pursuit of fundamental knowledge about the nature and behavior of living systems and the application of that knowledge to extend healthy life and reduce the burdens of illness and disability."

http://www.nih.gov/index.html

Johns Hopkins Medicine

"This virtual organization unites the physicians and scientists of The Johns Hopkins University School of Medicine with the health professionals and facilities that make up the broad

Johns Hopkins Health System."

http://www.hopkinsmedicine.org/

Mayo Clinic

"Mayo Clinic's web sites provide information and services from the world's first and largest integrated, not-for-profit group medical practice. Manage your health with information and tools that reflect the expertise of Mayo's 3,400 physicians and scientists, learn how to access medical services, and discover Mayo's medical research and education offerings."

http://www.mayoclinic.com/

WebMD

"Provides valuable health information, tools for managing your health, and support to those who seek information."

http://www.webmd.com/default.htm

PatientsLikeMe

"Our goal is to enable people to share information that can improve the lives of patients diagnosed with life-changing diseases. To make this happen, we've created a platform for collecting and sharing real world, outcome-based patient data and are establishing data-sharing partnerships with doctors, pharmaceutical and medical device companies, research organizations, and non-profits."

http://www.patientslikeme.com/

Appendix 10

Advocate Best Practices

You will face a series of emotional events while absorbing new medical and financial concepts. During this trying time, you will have to control your emotions to maintain your judgment.

Use a journal from day one to record facts, reminders, conversations, procedures and observations about your loved one's progress.

An effective advocate is a good listener. Ask questions and listen to doctors, nurses, caregivers and technicians to become a better advocate.

At the hospital, ask doctors nurses, caregivers and technicians about the topics and issues in this book and how they apply to your loved one. When discussing your loved one, always ask these two follow up questions:

"Are there any more questions I should be asking? Is there anything in addition that I should know?"

Ask doctors and nurses how you can be helpful and note it down. Be factual, specific, firm and clear in your communications with the hospital staff.

Be safety conscious at all times and ask about safety issues of newly acquired home healthcare equipment. Have equipment use, cleaning and maintenance demonstrated to you and follow recommended cleanliness and infection prevention measures.

Appendix 11

List Of Questions

Chapter 2 Before Leaving The Hospital: Questions To Ask Doctors And Nurses

Chapter 3   Before Leaving The Hospital: Arranging Visiting Nurses And Therapists

Chapter 5   Extra Equipment At Home

Chapter 8   Suction Machines
And Equipment Troubleshooting

**Chapter 9 Antibiotics And
Infection Prevention**

Chapter 10 Tube Feeding Issues And Tips

Index

A

B

Bacteria, 26, 145, 160-161, 163, 167-168, 172-174
Battery,
    digital blood pressure device, 49
    digital thermometer, 47
    electric patient lift, 93-94
    flashlights, 116
    portable suction machine, 150-151, 154-156
    smoke detector, 113
    tube feeding pump, 185, 194
Bed,
    manual, 82
    rails, 85, 176
    semi-electric, 80, 82-84, 86
    total electric, 83-84
Bedsores, 78, 87-89
Benefit Period (Medicare), 28-29
Billing issues, 213-215
Bladder infections, 163, 171-172, 174
Blood,
    glucose, 50
    laboratory analysis, 117, 122-123
    oxygen level, 37, 47-48, 133, 149
    pressure device, 32, 37, 49-50
    pressure, 37-38, 48, 49, 60
    thinner, 162
    transfusion, 29-30
    volume of sample, 128
Bloodstream connections, 15
Bowel movement, 39
Break away pants, 107
Breaths per minute, 38
Butterfly needle, 121

C

Call center, 221
Canula,
    tracheostomy, 43, 45, 60
    cuffed, cuffless, reusable, disposable, 44
    nasal, 138
Cap color (vacuum tube), 128

G

Gastric feeding tube, 193
Glaucoma, 33
Gloves, 42-43, 176
Glucometer, 50
Group administrator (insurance), 8, 218

H

Hand washing, 176
Handling yourself with doctors and nurses, 17
Hard stick, 121-122
Heart rate, 17, 37-38, 47-49, 60
HIPAA, 10
Home,
    health care department, 25, 63, 122, 129
    healthcare equipment troubleshooting,
        suction machines, 149
        tube feeding, 179, 194
    healthcare supply companies, 8, 219
        referrals, 52
Homebound, 4, 34, 55, 57-58, 64-65, 177
Home Health Agency (HHA), 59, 63, 65, 123
Home health aide, 59
Home healthcare bed,
    manual, 82
    semi-electric, 82
    total electric, 83
Home Healthcare Contact Information List, 8, 41, 222
Home healthcare medical devices, 32
Home healthcare supply companies, 8, 75, 219
Hospital,
    admission, 3
    dos and don'ts, 21
    exit examinations, 33
    free samples of disposables, 42
    Information List, 8
    isolation, 29
    laboratory, 122
    medical device non-emergency alerts, 15
    parking, 8, 20, 122

patient representative, 21
social worker, 21
stay, 1, 6, 27-28, 30, 36-37, 42, 117, 160
transport to, 3-5
Humidifier bottle,
mist machine, 142
oxygen concentrator, 137
Humidity display device, 145
Humidity (optimal), 139-140, 144-145

I

Immune system, 21, 168
Infection,
bladder, 26-27, 170, 172
intravenous (IV) line, 15
lung, 140, 169, 171
prevention, 27, 159, 175-177
repeating, 161
tube feeding precautions, 179
yeast, 163
Inhaled (medicines), 52, 171-172
Insurance,
additional information for claim processing,
197, 203-205, 211, 214-215, 218
companies, 115, 197-198, 214, 219
customer service agent, 218
customer service manager, 218
dealing with, 218-219
group administrator, 8, 218
nurse case manager, 218
primary, secondary, 198-200, 203
prompt payment laws, 219
re-instated, 9
Intensive Care Unit (ICU), 13-14
Intermittent catheterizing, 27, 32, 173-174
Intravenous (IV),
antibiotics, 162, 200
line, 14-16, 60, 121
medicines, 16, 52
pole, 185
Irregular heartbeat, 13

J

Jejunal feeding tube, 193
Journal, 38-40, 118-120, 124, 129, 135,
   137, 167, 170, 191, 217

L

LAL,
 See continuous low air loss mattress.
Laboratory,
 sample, 122-123, 128-130
 drop-off desk, 122
 hospital laboratory, 122, 129
 report, 62, 130, 162
Lancets (glucometer), 50
Learning to observe, 13
Leaving the hospital, 1, 31, 33, 57, 73
Liquids in/out, 39
Living Will, 7

M

Magnetic Resonance Imaging (MRI), 24
Massage, 131
Mattresses, 86
Mayo Clinic, 22
Medical,
 billing issues, 208, 213
 chart entries, 16, 19
 History, 5, 41
 necessity, 58, 77, 213
  certification of, 203-205, 212, 219
 Power of Attorney, 7
 records, 6-7, 9-10, 27, 41
Medicare,
 accept assignment, 51, 80
 allowed amount, 53, 80, 93, 201-205, 207, 212, 214
 appeal, 203, 212-213, 215
 card, 5
 certification for home visits, 123-124

N

National Institutes of Health (NIH), 22
Nebulizer, 80
Nebulized medicines, 171
Needle (butterfly), 121
Nose canula, 138, 143
Nurse,
    assignments, 18
    Assistant (CNA), 56
    call button, 14
    Licensed Vocational (LVN), 56, 58, 60
    Registered (RN), 18, 58, 60
    Practitioner (NP), 18

O

Occupational therapist (OT), 57, 59
On-board rechargeable battery, 93, 114-115, 185
Optimize care, 2
Over The Counter (OTC), 6, 41
Oximeter, 37, 47-48
Oxygen,
    bottle, 46, 134
        changing, 135
        common mistakes, 136-137
        face mask, 138, 143
        nose canula, 138, 143
        regulator and gauge, 134-137
        safety awareness, 137
        tracheal mask, 138, 143
        valve wrench, 134-136
    capped rental equipment (Medicare), 79-80
    concentrator, 46, 137-139, 141, 143
    troubleshooting connections, 139

P

Pacemaker, 5, 7, 24, 50
Pain, 35
Pain ruler, 35, 50-51

Paramedics, 4
Passy-Muir valve, 34, 45
Passive (range of motion) exercise, 65, 66
    See also active exercise.
Past Due, 197, 210-211
Patient lift, 73, 80, 91
    buying used, 94-95
    electric lift, 80, 92-94
    manual lift, 80, 92
    sling, 95
Patient,
    information forms, 6
    wristband, 7, 24
Pedaling machine, 67-68
Pharmacist, 164, 183, 186, 192
Phlebotomist, 121
Phone conversation tips, 219-222
Physical therapist (PT), 57
Physical therapy visits, 64
Physical therapy equipment, 57
Podiatrist, 34, 177
Pressure sores, 78, 87-89
Private ambulance, 4, 57
    medicare and insurance coverage, 4
Private billing companies, 215-216
Private duty nursing and caregiving, 56, 61
Private insurance, 5, 8, 109, 197-198, 211, 214
Provider, 200-202
Pulse oximeter, 37, 47-49
    blood oxygen saturation level, 47

Q

Quadriceps board, 67-68

R

Radiologist, 23
Radiologist's opinion, 55, 127
Recliner wheelchair, 96-99
Referrals, 52, 63
Rehabilitation (physical, speech, occupational), 64, 124, 126

Remote pacemaker testing, 50
Repeat hospital stays, 27
Replacement air filters, 147, 158
Research!America, 22
Resuming medicines at home, 36-37
Retail drug stores, 53
Returning to the hospital, 29
Room heater use and humidity, 140
Room (consumer) humidifiers, 143-145
    humistat, 144
    precautions, 145
Rounds, 19-20

S

Sanitizer gels, 176
Scooter, 78, 80-81, 111
Semi-electric bed, 82-84
Side effects, 5-6, 41, 160, 163-164, 166
Side Effects/Allergies List, 5-6, 41
Single occupancy room, 29
Skin, 16, 34, 60, 65, 86-87, 89, 102-103, 144, 173, 177
Smoke and CO detector, 109, 112-113
Speakers (audio), 126
Specialty pharmacy, 51-53, 192, 197
Speech therapist (ST), 57-59, 61, 64
Standing order, 62-63, 123, 153, 171
STAT, 63, 122-123
Stepladder, 116
Sterile saline, 153
Stethoscope, 42, 48-49
Styrofoam roller, 68
Suction machine, 46, 115, 149-152
    troubleshooting, 154-158
Supplemental oxygen,
    See oxygen.
Supplemental water, 179
Surgical masks, 21, 42

T

U

V

W

Walker, 77, 80, 111, 199
WebMD, 22
Wedge pillow, 90-91
Wheelchair,
    accessories, 99-106
    anti-tip bars, 99-100, 106, 111
    back cushion, 99-100
    basic, 80, 96-97
    headrest, 99-100
    leg extensions, 98-100
    motorized, 78, 80, 111
    ramps, 81, 99, 109-111
        safety, 111
    recliner, 96-99
    safety issues, 99
    seat belt, 1, 100, 102, 105, 111
    seat cushion, 99, 101-106
    tray, 67, 100, 105
White board, 118
Who pays first (Medicare or insurance), 199-200
Wound dressing creams, 43

X

X-rays, 23-24, 54
    See also mobile X-ray.

Y

Y Port tube feeding adapter, 45-46
Yankauer, 152